ADMINISTRATIVE THERAPY

TAVISTOCK

The International Behavioural and Social Sciences Library

MIND & MEDICINE
In 6 Volumes

ADMINISTRATIVE THERAPY

The Role of the Doctor in the Therapeutic Community

DAVID H CLARK

First published in 1964 by
Tavistock Publications (1959) Limited

Reprinted in 2001 by
Routledge
2 Park Square, Milton Park, Abingdon, Oxon, OX14 4RN
Simultaneously published in the USA and Canada
by Routledge
711 Third Avenue, New York, NY 10017

Routledge is an imprint of the Taylor & Francis Group, an informa business

Transferred to Digital Printing 2007

First issued in paperback 2013

© 1964 David H Clark

The publishers have made every effort to contact authors/copyright holders
of the works reprinted in the *International Behavioural and Social Sciences
Library*. This has not been possible in every case, however, and we would
welcome correspondence from those individuals/companies we have been
unable to trace.

These reprints are taken from original copies of each book. In many cases
the condition of these originals is not perfect. The publisher has gone to
great lengths to ensure the quality of these reprints, but wishes to point
out that certain characteristics of the original copies will, of necessity, be
apparent in reprints thereof.

British Library Cataloguing in Publication Data
A CIP catalogue record for this book
is available from the British Library

Administrative Therapy
ISBN 978-0-415-84585-4 (Pbk)
Mind & Medicine: 6 Volumes
ISBN 0-415-26512-6
The International Behavioural and Social Sciences Library
112 Volumes
ISBN 978-0-415-58414-2 (Set)

Administrative Therapy

THE ROLE OF THE DOCTOR
IN THE
THERAPEUTIC COMMUNITY

DAVID H. CLARK
F.R.C.P. Ed., D.P.M.

TAVISTOCK PUBLICATIONS

First published in Great Britain in 1964
by Tavistock Publications (1959) Limited
2 Park Square, Milton Park,
Abingdon, Oxon, OX14 4RN
in 11 point Times New Roman
by Ebenezer Baylis & Son Ltd
Worcester

CONTENTS

v

Contents

ACKNOWLEDGEMENTS

The greater part of this book was written in 1963, during the year of a Fellowship at the Center for Advanced Study in the Behavioral Sciences, Stanford, California, and I should like to record my gratitude to the Trustees of the Center and the Director, Ralph Tyler. Every clinician dreams of a chance to collate his experiences and reflect on them; to be given such an opportunity, to be transported to one of the most beautiful countries in the world and to be set down for a year in a community of reflective scholars, is an astounding boon and a wonderful privilege. I hope this book may offer some justification of the Center's generosity. I am grateful, too, to the Staff of the Center, to Preston Cutler, Jane Kielsmeier, Wayne Smith, and others for their support and kindness.

Acknowledgements are due, for permission to quote, to: Russell Sage Foundation, in respect of an extract from *From Custodial to Therapeutic Patient Care in Mental Hospitals* by M. Greenblatt, R. H. York, and E. L. Brown; Charles C. Thomas, Publisher, in respect of a passage from *Social Psychiatry in the Community, in Hospitals, and in Prisons* by Maxwell Jones; and to the World Health Organization in respect of excerpts from the Third Report of the Expert Committee on Mental Health *Technical Report Series*, No. 73, 1953.

The opinions here stated are my own, winnowed from the work of social psychiatry and therapeutic communities. They show, I hope, the influence of my teachers, especially Sir David Henderson and Dr S. H. Foulkes, and also of many friends and colleagues with whom I have discussed them, particularly, of course, Maxwell Jones. The individual chapters gained greatly from discussion held at the Center and I was helped by many comments, particularly, from David Hamburg, Harry Wilmer, Erich Lindemann, Jack Downing, David Daniels, and Frank Matsumoto.

Many other friends and colleagues also have given their assistance by reading drafts and proofs and offering critical comments. An administrative therapist should test all his projects, not least his books, by submitting them to discussion and criticism and gradually hammering them into something acceptable. It would in fact be most difficult adequately to thank all those who helped me in this way, particularly perhaps those whose advice I welcomed but did not always accept! But I am most grateful to them all. To my wife and family belong the credit for having provided, by their tolerance and encouragement, an atmosphere in which this book could grow.

My thanks are due to my secretaries on both sides of the Atlantic, Mrs Joan Warmbruun, Mr Graham Copeman, and Mrs Mary Mitchell for their help and patience.

But most of all I must record my debt to all those patients and colleagues who in our meetings over the years have taught me so much, never hesitating when necessary to point out my mistakes and failings. They have shared with me the excitements of exploring social psychiatry, of unlocking doors and tearing down railings, of opening communications and talking freely to one another, and they have borne with me as I learned painfully the task of administrative therapy. To all of them, but particularly to my friends, the patients, I must record my thanks, and it is to them, especially the patients of the long-stay wards of the mental hospital, that I dedicate this book.

INTRODUCTION

During the last twenty years institutional psychiatry has undergone numerous and profound changes. From being the medical officers of custodial institutions, concerned with security, with preventing escapes, and protecting society from their charges, psychiatrists have become the medical members of therapeutic communities, attempting to help and understand those placed in their care and to build a way of life that will help them soon to emerge as whole people.

This has involved many changes of attitude, many excursions into fields never regarded as medical. Traditional ways have been discarded and new nostrums tried, many of which have worked remarkably well. Those of us who have lived through this period know that we are doing work very different from that prescribed when we started, or from that which our seniors were then doing.

For some time there has seemed to me to be a need to set out what modern institutional psychiatry, especially that form of milieu therapy represented by the therapeutic community, demands of and promises to the doctor. This book is particularly designed for my colleagues who are coming into psychiatric institutions for the first time in the present exciting period and is designed as a handbook for the young doctor trying to understand and modify the world in which his patients live.

I have called it 'Administrative Therapy' because it combines two activities often seen as antagonistic, namely psychotherapy – the positive treatment of patients by psychological means – and administration – the daily business of planning, conferring, sitting on committees, and dealing with regulations and paperwork. I define administrative therapy as the art of treating patients in a psychiatric institution by administrative means or as the art of fulfilling the true doctor's role in a therapeutic community.

Something of this art was known to the great founders of institutional psychiatry such as Pinel, Tuke, Conolly, Browne, and Kirkbride. They had little doubt that the atmosphere of an institution could exert a beneficent influence on the patients in it and they called their work 'Moral Management'. As the nineteenth century passed, however, their work was forgotten, and until recently doctors thought of treatment – therapy – as something that was done exclusively for individual patients, preferably in a consulting-room or a sideroom off the ward, and of administration as a dreary, necessary process to which elderly psychiatrists addressed themselves and which had little bearing on the outcome of the patient's illness.

This view has been challenged and changed by the impact of the social sciences on the mental hospital and the development of milieu therapy.

The first chapter sketches the background and describes the observations of social scientists on it; the second mentions some of the experiments of the last twenty years; and the third outlines what seem to be principles underlying the organization of the therapeutic milieu.

In the fourth chapter the operations of administrative therapy are identified and explained; and in the fifth its application in three positions in the psychiatric hospital is set out. It is in these chapters that I present my main conclusions.

In the sixth chapter I examine certain characteristics helpful in administrative therapy and training that may be provided; and in the seventh I attempt further to define administrative therapy by discussing its relationship with other skills.

Finally, in Chapter Eight, the fact is discussed that little coherent theory exists as a base for practice, and points of development are indicated. As we get clearer theory and more validated results of administrative therapy, our practice will improve. In the meantime we have no choice. If we are to help our patients, we must change their drab world. To do this, we must practise administrative therapy. This book embodies what I have learnt about this important and hopeful development.

Administrative
Therapy

CHAPTER 1

The Mental Hospital and the Social Sciences

The background of the work to be discussed in this book is the mental hospital world of the 1930s. In that world all today's senior psychiatrists began their professional lives, into it came many of today's senior nursing staff as hopeful youngsters, and into it, as puzzled schizophrenic adolescents, came those who are now the shuffling, grey-faced automata of the back wards.

Scattered all over Western Europe and the United States were great institutions, remote from the towns, of antiquated architecture, little visited and little known to the general public except as places of dread mystery, names with which to frighten wayward children, a burden on the taxes, and the focus of occasional scandals. In them were hundreds – or thousands – of patients, a small underpaid staff of attendants, and a few doctors. They were places where little changed; they had an established way of operating which had been worked out over decades. The patients came in certified and resistant, obviously insane and rejected by their families; some died, some recovered and went out, but many remained for the rest of their lives; most of them remained

1

disorganized and 'mad' – either violent or lost in hallucinated apathy – though a number achieved a state of stable eccentricity and worked in the hospital departments. The small staff preserved order, prevented escapes, and saw that the patients were adequately fed and clothed; the hours were long, the pay low, and the work hard and occasionally dangerous; however, there were hospital houses, good sports facilities, a low retiring age, and a pension. Some staff were born on the estate, others came to work there, liked it, married another attendant, and settled; a complex web of intermarriages knit all the staff, nursing, maintenance, and clerical, together. The doctors examined the infrequent admissions, provided general medical care for patients and staff, and took responsibility for the running of the place. For them too, the pay was low and the work rather disheartening as there were no effective treatments and many patients remained chronically ill, but the pension was early and adequate, the rural setting and sports pleasant, and the doctor had a house and the perquisites of free vegetables and patients for domestic labour.

These hospitals were not always inefficient or unhappy places; the asylum cricket team was often famous, or the doctors' shooting parties; many of the better patients were well adjusted to a life of contented servitude, working as orderlies, storemen, or domestic servants in a cosier world than that outside. Among the younger doctors, too, there were those of energy and endeavour who conducted researches – innumerable post-mortems, or biochemical assays – or who made massive therapeutic onslaughts on the inert mass of misery confronting them, removing tonsils wholesale, or liberally dispensing thyroid extract.

This was the background, some details of which we shall soon discuss. The last thirty years have seen it change surprisingly. As it changed, doctors – the old doctors long entrenched, the young doctors just entering – have been called on to learn a new kind of medical work. It is this new work that this book discusses.

There were of course many vigorous, enthusiastic psychiatrists in the 1920s and 1930s but their energy found its scope outside the mental hospital. They left to work in outpatient clinics, or in private practice, following the exciting new developments in psychotherapy, in psycho-analysis or the physical treatments, for it was here that the future seemed to lie. They worked with individual patients, in the traditional medical consulting-room setting; this had been somewhat modified by the psycho-analytic methods of Freud, but these had if anything concentrated even further on the dyadic, one-doctor-one-patient relationship, even formally excluding the relatives and family from contact with the doctor. It was true that some psychiatrists, especially those working in the developing child guidance clinics with their powerful lady social workers, paid attention to the family setting; but even then the constant emphasis, as it was in most branches of medicine of that day, was on the individual patient and what was in his mind.

In the mental hospitals this traditional medical model was also accepted. The doctor carried out a 'mental examination' of the newly admitted patient; he made a diagnosis; he prescribed treatment and the nurses and attendants carried it out. This was proper doctoring; it was true that he had to spend time doing all sorts of 'administration' – answering letters of relatives, completing legal documents, censoring letters, finding satisfactory reasons for refusing the incessant requests to leave hospital, investigating allegations of patients and staff – but these things were not treatment, not proper doctoring.

B

3

Administrative Therapy

Towards the hundreds of 'chronic patients' the attitude was one of resignation. They were seen as suffering from incurable psychoses, mostly hereditary; there was little chance of their ever leaving hospital; the duty of the hospital and the doctor was to provide them with humane custody. 'After all, it is their home – they'll be here for the rest of their days – they can't help themselves, poor things.' Toward some of them, attachment, even friendship, could be developed; these were the quiet melancholics and paraphrenics who looked after the doctor's children or cultivated his garden; a joking relationship was comfortable with some of the deluded who would report each morning on the state of their influencing machines; but with many – the 'flexibilitas' cases who stood statue-like in a puddle of their own urine for days, weeks, and years on end, the catatonics with their wild outbursts of dangerous violence, the 'caution' patients who were forever attempting bizarre self-mutilation, little contact was possible and the doctor could only attempt to limit the physical damage to the patient and to those about him. A certain amount of personal danger and of involvement in degradation and brutality were accepted as inevitable if regrettable aspects of mental hospital work.

The doctor in the mental hospital was in a dilemma. He found himself working in a place where many patients did not get better; he had to endorse many things – such as straitjackets, padded cells, forced feeding – which he did not like and which conflicted with his picture of himself as a beneficent healer; yet he could see no other alternative. The repugnant ward rituals were deeply established and entrenched and any attempt by a young doctor to change them was effectively defeated by the senior nursing staff of the ward. Nearly every young doctor made an attempt to change things and found himself impotent. It was like beating his head against a brick wall; even the patients seemed to prefer the *status quo*. Most able and sensitive doctors either left the hospital and went into private practice, or accepted the situation and made the best of it by becoming superintendents and interesting themselves in buildings, farms, committee work, medical politics, or forensic psychiatry. Only the defeated stayed on the wards indefinitely and they retreated into formal medical activity. The doctors did not like their hospitals much but they knew nothing better. As far as the doctor could tell, things had always been this way; in the reminiscences of the most senior staff members or the oldest patient, stretching back at least fifty years into the youth of his grandfather, things had always been much the same. It was a strange special world which dealt in misery and degradation made tolerable by rural surroundings; his was a dreary but necessary and fairly honourable calling.

The first break into this static world came with the physical treatments – insulin coma therapy in the mid 1930s, convulsion therapy, first with cardiazol and then with electricity, in the early 1940s. These treatments made a tremendous change in the atmosphere of the hospitals. The doctors, the nurses, and the attendants could all feel they were really *doing* something; many patients made dramatic recoveries from years of withdrawal. A wind of enthusiasm – which at times rose to a tornado of *furor therapeuticus* – swept through the hospitals. These methods were, however, still *individual* therapy. The patients were assessed individually, chosen on the basis of their symptoms, and treated personally. The organization of the treatment unit, or the rehabilitation programme, was only a necessary administrative exercise. It was during the 1950s, and during the arguments over the significance of widespread application of tranquillizers, that explicit notice

5

began to be taken of the milieu in which treatment was taking place. Gradually some psychiatrists began to suspect that this might be more important than the 'treatment' around which it was organized.

This is seen strikingly in the story of insulin coma therapy. Introduced by Sakel in 1935, it was widely adopted as a form of treatment for patients suffering from schizophrenia. Many chronically ill patients, given up as hopeless, made dramatic recoveries; many acutely ill patients recovered far quicker than was expected. Because it was a dangerous and occasionally fatal treatment, a well-organized and highly trained staff team was necessary. Many hospitals set up an 'insulin unit'; because this was often the most exciting and rewarding section of the hospital, it attracted the keen, eager, well-qualified young doctors, nurses, and attendants. They formed tightly knit teams, working together through crises and long dramas of life-saving so that they came to know and trust one another as colleagues and comrades. The patients were mostly young schizophrenics with changing symptomatology; though often very disturbed, they were accessible and emotionally open, so that warm relationships sprang up. To a visitor it was striking how different the relationships in a good insulin unit were from the rest of the hospital. The staff were on easy, confident terms with one another, with private jokes and a special jargon; the patients were spoken to warmly by their Christian names, spoon-fed, and encouraged; all played games together in the afternoon, patients, nurses, and even doctors. But little of this was mentioned in the publications, which still discussed varieties of insulin, dosages, potentiators, frequency and depth of comas, symptomatic prognosticators, and such individual, unemotional 'objective' considerations. This treatment continued in vogue for nearly twenty years, despite a few critical voices. Then Bourne[9] voiced the growing challenge and Ackner, Harris and Oldham,[1] in a classic study, showed that whatever the effective agent was, it was not the insulin. Attention then turned to the intensive group experiences provided in an insulin unit and the possibility of understanding and using them.

The dawning appreciation of the importance of social factors in treatment procedures come partly from the general expansion of interest in the social sciences which occurred in the post-war period and which began to penetrate the private world of the mental hospitals in the 1950s.

The social sciences are a comparatively modern growth. Though a few sociologists were writing in the nineteenth century, it was not until the 1920s and 1930s that social psychology and social anthropology emerged as distinct disciplines with a growing body of theory. The experiences of the Second World War made many thinking men acutely aware of social factors in human life, in labour relations, in army training, in prisoner-of-war camps, and many other fields. A number of popular books on anthropology, social psychology, and industrial sociology, especially the 'human relations' school, were widely read (see Reading List, p. 151). They looked at human institutions as a mesh of personal relationships modified by tradition forming a 'culture' that was most powerful in its effects on the individual. They carried the idea that the way in which people lived, the culture in which they were immersed, had important effects on how they behaved, and that many ways of behaving previously accepted as basic human characteristics were not seen in some cultures. They suggested that perhaps the way in which the

7

mental hospital was organized had something to do with the behaviour of the people in it, and that it might be possible to look at mental hospital life and work in a new way. Gradually, studies have appeared which have taught the doctors a great deal about the life of their institutions and some of the effects that they had on the people in them.

Rowland,[46,47] in 1938, commented on state hospital life, its interactions and friendship patterns. Bateman and Dunham,[5] in 1948, stated firmly that the 'employee culture' with its custodial pessimism was a factor working against patients' discharge. The material from which these conclusions were drawn was not published until 1960 by Dunham and Weinberg;[20] this is a careful factual description of the life of Columbus State Hospital, Ohio, in the immediate post-war period and is one of the most useful permanent records of the way of life of the custodial state hospital.

The studies which had the greatest impact, however, were those of Stanton and Schwartz.[51] Stanton, a psychiatrist, and Schwartz, a social psychologist, worked together for three years at Chestnut Lodge Sanitarium, Maryland. This was a most exceptional institution – a small, private hospital devoted to the psycho-analytic treatment of psychotic patients; each patient had an hour's psycho-analysis daily and since the fees were about $12,000 (£4,000 sterling) per year, most patients came from a privileged background. The studies, however, were illuminating to all who worked in psychiatric institutions.

Although they described some interesting findings, particularly the 'triangular conflict', their major contribution was their way of looking at the hospital as a total culture. They looked at all the people, the patients, the attendants, the nurses, and the doctors, as people living and working together, sharing certain assumptions, and reacting to one

8

another. They gathered their material by sitting in staff meetings and discussions, by sitting on the wards for hours to note what happened, and by correlating and analysing their observations. They emphasized how events in one area affected others. They described how budgetary problems had forced the director to call for pressure on certain patients to pay their bills; how this had annoyed the senior doctors; how this had reverberated through the residents and the nurses and culminated in a series of violent episodes on the locked ward. In a series of ward observations they investigated how the staff responded to patients; the staff believed that they gave or should give attention to the patients that needed it most, that is, the withdrawn, mute, and helpless patients, and that they should discourage the attention-seeking patients. One study showed the reverse to be true; the importunate patient received the things she demanded, while the withdrawn patient discouraged the nurse by her negativism and received even less than before.

Their analysis of 'triangular conflict' started from a not uncommon mental hospital situation – a crisis of mounting hospital concern about a disturbed demanding patient and a staff member who had 'become too involved'. All hospitals have these crises occasionally; they cause great concern and anxiety to all the staff, especially to nursing and medical administrators and teachers. The crisis often ends badly and sometimes tragically. The staff member involved, often one of the keenest or most sensitive of the doctors or nurses, is severely demoralized, and usually leaves the hospital and often the profession.

The traditional view of this situation had been in terms of individual psychology – the malignancy of the patient's illness, the personality flaws of the doctor or nurse, the value of thorough training in preventing 'unhealthy involvement' in the emotional problems of patients. Stanton and Schwartz showed that, relevant though these were, the situation was essentially a social one, involving many other staff but especially one other key figure – a staff member of approximately equal rank to the central staff member. The two protagonists might be two nurses, two doctors, a doctor and a nurse. These and the patient formed the triangle. The problem had begun much earlier when the two staff members disagreed about the proper plan of treatment for the patient. Each thought the other was wrong but they did not say so openly; they did not, or could not, talk about it, and what contact they had began to dissolve; they avoided one another, often 'accidentally'; appointments were not kept and messages not delivered. The problem became worse and the patient more distraught and demanding; the two protagonists more active but less in contact. Other staff members and superiors were involved in the outbursts and crises and began to express opinions; there was muttering in corners and shaking of heads. One of the original two became isolated and came to feel that only he understood the patient; everyone else was wrong, punitive, muddleheaded, formalistic, or unkind. He spent extra hours and evenings on the ward in 'special sessions' with the patient, and began to show increasing signs of personal stress – agitation, insomnia, overactivity – until the final break came. They pointed out that this usually took the form of an attack, verbal or physical, on the patient by the staff member. This was followed by acute shame and guilt and the final collapse of the staff member, who usually sought his superior, resigned from his work, and sought personal analysis or some completely different type of work.

On the basis of this social analysis, they propounded a solution which experience has proved effective – a confrontation, fairly early in the process, of the two staff members, in which they talk openly, discuss their differences, face, and, if possible, resolve them. Finally, they work out a plan of treatment and behaviour in which their respective parts and responsibilities are clear and which they can both openly endorse. This contains the crisis, brings effective treatment to the patient, and saves the isolated staff member. In units where this lesson has been fully learned, whenever a patient looks like becoming a 'special case' the staff ask themselves where the covert disagreement lies and take steps to resolve it. This has proved an effective tool of social therapy.

Caudill,[13] a social anthropologist, entered a small neurosis unit as a 'patient'; he lived there for some months and described what happened to him. He sets out the way in which a patient is taught his role; the other patients instruct him on how a patient should behave, not only by what they do, but also quite openly in discussions round the fire in the evenings; they tell him what sorts of fantasies each doctor likes to hear during psychotherapy, what sort of behaviour will win a weekend pass or permission to shave, and what are the transgressions that will bring reprisals. Later Caudill returned to the hospital without disguise as an observer and wrote up further observations in a book[12] which is another useful demonstration of what the social scientist can tell the doctors.

None of these, however, was an ordinary mental hospital. Belknap,[6] a Texas sociologist, carried out a survey of a typical state hospital which remains the classic study of the unmodified traditional mental hospital culture. He started from the striking historical fact that this hospital had been 'reformed' a number of times; following scandals, the people in charge had been sacked and new administrators appointed – only to have the cycle repeated a few decades later. He analysed the length of time people stayed in the hospital.

Administrative Therapy

The patients, of course, stayed longest; but he showed that doctors and administrative nurses were transitory members of the hospital; the only really stable staff were a nuclear group of attendants and maintenance employees who spent their entire working lives in the institution. He found that these people controlled the wards and the details of the patients' daily lives, and were in fact the carriers of the enduring culture of the institution. He analysed the structure of a typical back ward, and described how it operated; he set out the status layers and showed that there was a stratified society with six layers – the doctors; the charge attendant and his deputies; the attendants; the worker (*élite*) patients; the limited privilege patients; and finally those patients without any privileges at all. He pointed out that everyone, however psychotic, knew where he stood on this scale and showed an awareness of his rights and obligations. He showed that this was the enduring reality of the mental hospital; that this back-ward life of long-stay patients and long-stay attendants was what persisted, while head nurses, medical directors, nursing supervisors, occupational therapists, and others came and went. He then examined the beliefs of these attendants – Dunham's 'employee culture'; he showed that it was humane, custodial, and pessimistic; they believed that patients were unlikely to leave hospital and that if they did they would probably just have to return; they accepted that their work was despised and that supplies would always be short; they accepted the need to use coercion to maintain control but they were mostly well disposed to their patients and tried to make their life as comfortable as possible.

Goffman, a sociologist who had made a number of interesting studies of people in unusual situations (e.g. confidence tricksters placating their victims) and who writes with a vivid twist of the pen, spent a year at St Elizabeth's

Hospital, Washington, D.C. He wrote several articles, the first of which appeared in 1957[25] and then collected them in a book.[26] Goffman sees the world as a place where man is constantly under the attack of unfriendly forces which he must evade, placate, or fight. In 'The Underlife of a Public Institution; A Study of Ways of Making Out in a Mental Hospital', he describes how a vast federal mental hospital bears down on the individual patient and the constant shifts he is put to. It brings home to the doctor who has buttressed himself with the picture of his hospital as a primarily beneficent and therapeutic institution how it may appear to a perceptive but critical observer. But Goffman goes much more deeply into the social processes behind the behaviour he so vividly depicts and points out much of its inevitability and social utility.

He analyses mental hospitals along with other 'total institutions' – monasteries, prisons, boarding schools, and officers' academies. He points out that all these institutions develop certain social patterns – a psychological isolation from the outside world; a denial of previous social or educational differences; a 'stripping process' in which the entrant loses all those things that gave him his previous identity (clothes, money, personal belongings, hair) and is dressed in uniform garb; a private jargon; a unique and peculiar system of rewards and punishments for actions not regarded as exceptional in the outside world; a system of special roles such as 'court jester'; and special Saturnalia-like festivals. In 'The Medical Model and Mental Hospitalization: Some Notes on the Vicissitudes of the Tinkering Trades', he points out how medical dogmatism, which works so well in normal society when the patient is free to accept or reject the doctor's advice, has unexpected results in the mental hospital where the patient is completely within the doctor's control. He has

13

shed a great deal of valuable, though uncomfortable, light on the life of the mental hospital.

Other studies have described the deleterious effect that long years of incarceration in an institution have on people. Notable were Martin's[36] article describing 'Institutionalization' and Barton's[3] booklet, *Institutional Neurosis*. Both contended that many of the 'signs' of chronic schizophrenia were the product of long years of regimented institutional living deprived of personal belongings, outside contacts, or any stimuli other than repressive ones. Barton mentions apathy, lack of initiative, loss of interest, deterioration in personal habits, toilet, and general standards; he describes a characteristic posture, 'the hands held across the body or behind an apron, the shoulders drooped, the head held forward. The gait has a shuffling quality, movements at the pelvis and knees are restricted, although physical examination shows a full range of movement at these joints'.

All these studies have illuminated the traditional custodial mental hospital structure. They have shown that it does grave harm to the patients by increasing their social withdrawal, their dependence, and their crippledom, and they have suggested that much of what we saw in the 'typical back-ward chronic' was the result, not of his schizophrenia, but of the way he had been 'looked after' for several decades.

We next consider some of the attempts to apply these insights and to help patients by restructuring the milieu in which they live.

CHAPTER 2

Milieu Therapies

During the years when social scientists were beginning to illuminate the murky world of the mental hospitals with their comments, a number of psychiatrists were trying to improve the state of the patients committed to their care by changing the life of the institutions. These attempts, empirically developed, and more often based on humane conviction than on psychological theory, were the beginnings of administrative therapy.

Ever since the first days of institutional psychiatry there had been attempts to structure the institutions to produce desired results in the inmates. Some won favour and were then forgotten, like the Moral Treatment of the first half of the nineteenth century; some made a permanent contribution to psychiatric practice, like Conolly's No Restraint Method, which set a limit to coercion which, despite backslidings, has never been forgotten; others, after a vogue, were discredited, like Weir Mitchell's Bed Rest Treatment.

Only the systems of recent years will be discussed here. Three stand out: Work Therapy, Open Doors, and Therapeutic Communities. They were interdependent, and an administrative therapist developing one usually found himself involved with the others. Out of them and the attempts to

15

assess and understand them have developed what we know as Milieu Therapy and Administrative Therapy.

WORK THERAPY

The roots of modern work therapy go back to Dr Hermann Simon[49] of Guetersloh Hospital in Germany, who developed a régime based on work with Teutonic vigour and enthusiasm. Visits to his hospital inspired psychiatrists, the Dutch especially, so that Dutch mental hospitals for the last thirty years have demonstrated how much work severely impaired persons can do and how this prevents a great deal of the deterioration and degradation considered an essential part of mental illness.

Dutch mental hospitals contain mostly long-stay patients, and they are expected to work to help to support the hospital. The hospitals have patients doing not only the usual maintenance tasks – farming, housework, labouring – but also many industrial tasks. They make army equipment, undertake electrical assembly work, and manufacture clothing and footwear for commercial sale. Work must be properly finished and spoiled work is not tolerated. The whole atmosphere is authoritarian and the patients' rewards are nominal; there is little attempt to explore or harness social dynamic forces. But nevertheless the achievement is striking; there are no wards full of idle, deteriorated, neglected, hopeless persons; there are few incontinent patients, no patients half naked and in tattered clothing, very few persons showing catatonic immobility and flexibilitas cerea, and few restraint devices.

In 1933 the English Board of Control was arranging for English psychiatrists to visit Holland, and the development of occupational therapy in British mental hospitals dates mostly from that time. There was, of course, a tendency for it to be confined only to the better patients. To organize work for the more sick patients was more difficult.

Dr T. P. Rees of Warlingham Park told how he ordered a nurse to take a group of refractory ward patients out to clear some woodland. The man refused, saying that the patients were violent, and that a pension would be little use to his widow. Dr Rees discharged the man summarily, shouldered an axe and led the party into the wood himself.

Carstairs, Clark, and O'Connor,[10] in a post-war visit to European hospitals, described how the Dutch had greatly extended industrial work in hospitals. Factories were started in English mental hospitals, at Banstead Hospital London, (Carstairs, O'Connor, and Raunsley,[11] Baker[2]), at Cheadle Royal Hospital, Manchester (Wadsworth[53,54]), and at Glenside Hospital, Bristol (Early[21] [22]). In each case there were considerable organizational difficulties to overcome, financial and marketing arrangements to make, and manufacturers and trade unionists to convince.

After the factory work at Glenside Hospital, Bristol, had reached a certain level, Dr Early wished to extend it outside. He found that this was difficult and very slow within the complexities of the finances of the National Health Service. He had by now a number of contacts among Bristol business men whose altruism was excited by the chance to help the long-stay patients. With their help he set up the Industrial Therapy Organization (Bristol) with two bishops and a lord mayor on its board. They rented an abandoned school, hired staff, and set up a small factory, with several routine tasks, especially assembling

17

ballpoint pens: all the money went to the patients. The project prospered. Many patients from the hospital were employed and some moved on to independent life. Other schemes were operated such as a highly successful drive-in car-wash. Articles were published[21] [22] and a film of the project made. There were of course difficulties. Local trade unionists asked questions, wondering if there was exploitation of the patients. Dr Early went and talked to representatives of the Trades Council, who visited the industrial departments in the hospital. They were entirely won over and were so impressed that they commended the scheme to other employers and arranged for the Secretary of the national Trade Union Congress to visit the factory and endorse the project.

All this involved Dr Early in much 'non-medical' activity, from negotiating rates of pay to interviewing bishops. But he had accepted one of the basic propositions of administrative therapy – that if a doctor wishes to use social psychiatry effectively to help his patients he must be prepared to undertake many tasks that are not usually regarded as the business of doctors.

By 1962 there were some 60 industrial workshops in English mental hospitals and many patients earning money. Similar projects were developing in Veterans Administration hospitals in the United States. These workshops are important in giving meaning and manifest monetary value to a patient's activity, but to achieve them called for much non-medical activity by doctors.

OPEN DOORS

The degrading devices employed to restrain furious lunatics have always filled compassionate physicians with dismay, and many have cherished the memory of Pinel and the famous picture in which he is seen striking the chains off the patients in the Bicêtre, even when their daily work forced them to condone something very different.

In the century and a half since Pinel and the century since Conolly, the standards of care of the mentally ill in Britain had been gradually raised to a fairly humane level by the constant vigilance of the Commissioners in Lunacy and their successors of the Board of Control. But in 1945 the majority of patients were still locked up and denied many liberties.

Dr George Macdonald Bell always hated having to lock people up. In describing the first time he as a junior assistant medical officer had to assist in putting a patient into a padded cell, he says, 'I resolved then that either I must leave psychiatry or change it.' He became Superintendent of Dingleton Hospital, Melrose, Scotland, a 400-bed county hospital, and began to press for Open Doors. Though he used persuasion to overcome the fears of his staff, he had no hesitation in ordering the changes. In 1949 the last door of the hospital was opened, and since that time no patient in Dingleton has been locked up. There were many anxieties and difficulties, especially with the local townsfolk, and Dr Bell spent many hours with the local police, the bailies, the provost, the lawyers, and the citizens cajoling and explaining. He had to appear in court to explain the freedom given to patients who had broken the law. But gradually he won over the staff of the hospital and the burghers of Melrose until they are all proud of their hospital and what it does.

The idea that mental hospital ward doors could be open spread gradually. In 1953 Dr Duncan Macmillan opened the last ward door at Mapperley Hospital, Nottingham. In London, Dr T. P. Rees, who had been active in developing work therapy, took a leading part in opening ward doors and promoting discussion of the issue. During the later 1950s there was much argument in British psychiatry about the possibility and desirability of open doors. This coincided with the widespread introduction of the tranquillizing drugs, which undoubtedly made the change less difficult because many patients were not so acutely disturbed. But the drugs and the freedom helped each other; the first open doors (at Dingleton) were long before the tranquillizers. Gradually hospitals opened most of their ward doors and by 1963 some 80 per cent of English psychiatric patients were in open wards; in some hospitals a few locked wards were maintained but in a number of hospitals all the doors were open. The advantages for the patients and staff were striking; tension disappeared, violence declined, 'escapes' were no longer a problem, the staff were able to give their attention to therapy rather than custody. But the process of change had involved many doctors in an exercise in administrative therapy; within the hospital they had to persuade the staff of the desirability of changing long-held practices and to allay their anxieties; outside the hospital they had to meet civic leaders and anxious groups of householders and win their support.

At Fulbourn Hospital three long-stay workers' wards were opened in 1951. In 1954, after setting up a full activity programme for the other patients, we began cautiously to open further ward doors. There were full staff discussions first; some were for it, others against. They recalled that for years any nurse allowing a patient to escape was summarily dismissed and inquired what the position would be now – 'Who would take the can back?' – I said that we decided this change together; if there was trouble I would accept the blame. We opened the doors of a ward of long-stay paranoid women; nothing untoward happened, though several patients commented unfavourably that now the other people could get in.

The nurses found great relief at no longer having to run to and fro unlocking doors and counting people; other ward charge nurses asked permission to unlock their wards. During this time I spent many evenings talking to Rotary Clubs, Townswomen's Guilds, Mothers' Unions, and Parent-Teacher Associations about what we were doing. Again and again I emphasized the benefits of freedom for the mentally sick, and reassured them that no person regarded as dangerous would be allowed out unchecked. I spoke especially to our neighbouring villages and asked them to report any untoward incidents, which they helpfully did.

Within the hospital we were still experimenting and did not know how far we could go. My own doubts are preserved in an address I gave in October 1955[15] in which I said I thought that a hospital near a large centre of population could not work with entirely open doors.

As we experimented with freedom, however, we became more and more impressed by its value for the patients. By 1956 all wards were open except the last two, where all the most disturbed and troubling patients were gathered. We had many more discussions; we realized that some of these patients could not have full liberty, but that the locked door was harmful to the rest of the ward. By arranging intensive nursing of these patients it was possible to allow the nurses to open the doors of the 'disturbed wards', at first hesitantly and then with increasing confidence. The nurse in charge was allowed to lock the ward door temporarily if it seemed essential, but this was done less and less often. In 1958 the last permanently locked door was opened. Though there are always a few patients for whom intensive nursing and surveillance are necessary, it has never been necessary to return to permanently locked doors and the open-door hospital has become a matter of pride to all members of the staff, so that they wrote articles describing it.[42]

Here again, however, I was involved in a great deal of 'non-medical' activity; within the hospital in taking the chair at prolonged and anxious discussions of policy, and outside the hospital in lecturing to civic groups, talking to policemen, giving interviews to the press and radio, and answering phone calls from the anxious.

The development of open doors in the United States has been slower and the same controversies are exercising American psychiatrists in the 1960s as concerned the English in the 1950s. They have greater difficulties; the hospitals are larger; there are probably more violent persons committed to state hospitals; public opinion is not so favourable. Nevertheless, St Laurence State Hospital, New York, has had all its doors open for some years, and many ward doors are gradually being opened.

THERAPEUTIC COMMUNITIES

In the late 1920s, Harry Stack Sullivan organized a unit for what he called 'modified psycho-analytic treatment of schizophrenics' at the Sheppard and Enoch Pratt Hospital in Maryland. This did not receive a great deal of notice, perhaps because of the dramatic development of insulin coma therapy shortly after, but in retrospect can be seen as one of the first therapeutic communities. The unit was for six male patients with a staff of six young attendants whom he indoctrinated personally and it is clear that they managed to develop an intensive atmosphere of warmth and acceptance. His original articles were reprinted in 1962 in a book,[52] which also contained two memoirs that give a picture of the atmosphere Sullivan created and the intense personal interest he devoted to it.

In 1939 Myerson[39] published an account of the 'Total Push' method of treatment which he had worked out. He appears to have started from the observation that long-stay patients improve if someone gives them intensive attention; he reasoned that the more they had, the better they would do, and he arranged to bring everyone – occupational therapists, domestics, nurses, attendants, doctors, in on the business of keeping the patient active. There have been few further publications about this method but the striking name has never been forgotten. As we have learned more we have realized that pushing people makes them resistant and that personality growth needs more subtle encouragement. However, his work was a reminder of the striking initial results seen in neglected people by mere vigour and enthusiasm alone.

None of these beginnings, however, gained major attention. Psychiatrists in the 1930s were involved in individual psychotherapy or else caught up in the flood of therapeutic enthusiasm flowing from the physical treatments. Army experience during the Second World War, however, reminded psychiatrists of the immense influence of group and social factors on the individual's health, and a number of British psychiatrists began to explore the possibilities of using these social forces positively, particularly at Northfield Hospital, an English unit for soldiers suffering from psychoneurotic disorders.

Administrative Therapy

Bion and Rickman[8] took a group of these demoralized men and directed their attention from their individual anxieties to those of their group, insisting on their taking responsibility for the organization of the ward. This experiment, though short, indicated the way in which social restructuring might help individual difficulties. The reaction of the senior N.C.O.s and the commanding officer were also prophetic of the difficulties which many administrative therapists were later to face.

Foulkes worked at Northfield at a later stage; his first book[23] is mostly concerned with small group treatment but also describes the use of the environment by a sensitive psychotherapist. He speaks of adjourning a group session to attend a ward football match, discusses the therapeutic effect of being a member of a successful dance band, and stresses the importance of examining and affecting the way that patients are together.

The 'Northfield group' of British social psychiatrists contributed a number of papers to an issue of the *Bulletin of the Menninger Clinic* (1946). Notable was one by Main[34] in which he drew attention to the damage that the traditional hospital does to the dependent neurotic personality in a series of vivid phrases ('the medical man educated to play a grandiose role among the sick', 'the fine traditional mixture of charity and discipline they receive is a practised technique for removing their initiative as adult beings and making them "patients" '). He called for the organization of hospitals that would cure rather than damage neurotics. It was in this article that the phrase 'therapeutic community' was first employed.

Maxwell Jones was one of the most significant figures throughout this period in developing therapeutic communities for the treatment of disordered people, and the idea is

24

now closely linked with his name. He started community work during the war with cardiac neurotics and continued with a rehabilitation unit for returned prisoners-of-war. In 1947 he opened an Industrial Neurosis Unit in a wing of Belmont Hospital, Surrey, at first for those with long histories of unemployment and later for 'psychopaths' of all kinds (in 1954 the name was changed to Social Rehabilitation Unit). In his first book[29] he described these communities. The pattern of activity at the Belmont Unit changed over the years; for example, psychodrama was much used in the earlier years but was later abandoned. But social therapy was always paramount; although work with individual patients continued, the main therapeutic work was in the meetings – the daily community meetings, the group meetings, the workshop meetings – and everything that happened was examined. Because it was recognized that the main difficulty of these patients lay in their social relationships, these were constantly examined and studied; incidents in the ward and the workshop were discussed and analysed at length.

This unit was strikingly different from any previous psychiatric institution. Traditional marks of status were abandoned; no uniforms were worn and everyone was addressed by Christian names. The Unit welcomed visitors for whom it provided an exhilarating and perplexing experience of a place where everyone joined in vigorous and uninhibited discussion of behaviour and attitudes.

Maxwell Jones's impact, however, was not only in the work at the Unit, nor in his writings, but in his personal influence as a consultant and visiting lecturer to hospitals and groups in Britain and the United States, where many psychiatrists and other workers were first dramatically introduced to the idea that patients could help one another, that staff relationships need not always be rigid and formalized, and that the environment, imaginatively reconstructed, could powerfully aid a patient's recovery.

The work of the Belmont Unit was studied by Rapoport and his team of social scientists, who published their findings in 1960.[44] They described the culture that was by then established with its group meetings and constant self-examination. They described how this culture affected the patients with their long personal history of psychopathic and antisocial behaviour, and analysed some of the results achieved. They also discussed the effects the culture had on the staff, especially those with professional trainings, the doctors, nurses, and social workers. They distinguished certain cultural themes – democratization, permissiveness, communalism, and reality confrontation – and the implications and internal contradictions of these. They felt that the value of the Unit to the patients was to some extent affected by a tendency to develop a very special culture and to value adjustment to the Unit culture rather higher than eventual adjustment to the culture and standards of the outside world – to which the patients, and even the staff, must ultimately return.

In 1953 the World Health Organization published the third report of its Expert Committee on Mental Health.[59] Among the Committee were Kraus of Sandpoort, Holland, Rees of Warlingham Park, England, and Sivadon of Neuilly-sur-Marne, France, each a superintendent of a first-class hospital, a leader in his own country, and an outstanding administrative therapist.

In a chapter on 'The Community Mental Hospital' the Committee discuss the atmosphere of the mental hospital which was considered 'the most important single factor in the efficacy of the treatment given'. They then set out some of the essential constituents of this atmosphere – that the patient's individuality should be preserved, that patients should be assumed to be trustworthy, that good behaviour should be encouraged, that patients should be assumed to be capable of responsibility and initiative, and that there should be a programme of planned, purposeful activity.

This report shows how far thinking had advanced by 1953. The following years were taken up with the difficult task of working these principles out in practice, in spreading the work and maintaining it.

American interest began to grow and there have been a number of publications describing programmes.

In 1955 Greenblatt, York, and Brown[27] published a detailed account of the changes which had been made in Boston Psychopathic Hospital, in Bedford Veterans Administration Hospital, and in Metropolitan State Hospital, all in the Boston area of Massachusetts. Boston Psychopathic Hospital, though an outstanding teaching and research institution, had had oppressive and squalid conditions on its back wards. Under the leadership of Dr Harry C. Solomon it had been changed into a lively, hopeful, active place with greatly increased contributions from and freedom for the patients, the attendances and the lower-ranking staff. Similar changes had occurred in the other two hospitals. In the introduction they suggest three working hypotheses of the work described.

1. The basic function of the mental hospital 'is the utilization of every form of treatment available for restoring patients to health and helping them improve sufficiently to be able to leave the hospital at the earliest possible moment; and short of such success, it is aiding them to live as nearly normal lives as possible within the institutional setting . . .'

2. 'The utilization of *every* form of therapy available

requires planned and systematic use of the whole environment, consisting of both physical resources and social interaction between all categories of staff and patients . . .'

3. 'For purposes of making effective use of the social environment of the hospital, including improvements of the motivation of personnel, concepts and methods of research developed by the behavioural sciences should be tested and utilized wherever feasible.'

By this time interest in the use of the social structure in treatment was widespread and many experiments were going on. A conference in Boston in 1956 brought many of the leading workers together and their papers were later published.[28] These papers with those at two later conferences, in 1957 at the Walter Reed Army Institute of Research[55] and in New York in 1959,[19] constitute a valuable collection of accounts of therapeutic community experiments, of explorations, and of studies in the field. In more recent years the approach has been tried in many mental hospitals, in Britain, in the United States, and in other countries. There have been many brief articles descriptive of programmes limited to wards and units. The adequate description of any social process, however, is an exacting task. The greater the cast, the wider the canvas, the more difficult is description. It is probably for this reason that there are few accounts of total programmes.

Wilmer, who had worked with Maxwell Jones, organized a therapeutic community in a Navy admitting ward in Oakland, California.[56] It was a 34-bed ward receiving acute admissions and holding them for up to ten days. The unit had previously used the standard methods of control – seclusion, sedation, and coercion. Wilmer set up a community meeting every morning followed by a staff meeting. In these he analysed and examined all the happenings of a stormy ward; the patients began to help their confused comrades effectively and to 'wise them up' in a helpful rather than the traditional hostile way. Seclusion became unnecessary and sedation fell markedly.

As the staff came to trust him, there were lengthy discussions of the tensions and anxiety of the enlisted corpsman attempting to care for deeply disturbed and often dangerous patients. As the ward developed its special culture, they had to include the night-duty staff and the other doctors of the hospital. Many problems arose and were overcome and the morale of the unit was high. The story was later dramatized and filmed ('People need People'). Wilmer's story is an outstanding account of a successful therapeutic community which shows a good deal of effective administrative therapy.

In England during the 1950s Martin had been developing therapeutic communities at Claybury Hospital. He started with a mixed neurosis unit in an outlying villa but later developed further communities in the admitting and long-stay wards of the hospital. He describes the ten years of change in a book[37] designed for lay as well as professional readers. This gives a clear picture of the changes and the humane Christian philosophy in forming them but unfortunately gives very little picture of the key role played by Martin himself as senior psychiatrist in charge of the unit. As the concepts spread through Claybury Hospital, all came to accept the principle he propounded that 'a therapeutic community is one in which a deliberate effort is made to use to the fullest possible extent in a comprehensive treatment plan the contributions of all staff and patients'.

SOCIAL PSYCHIATRY

During all this period the general concept of social psychiatry

29

was developing and expanding, and psychiatrists were looking beyond the personal problems presented by their patients into their families, their workshops and the societies in which they lived. Epidemiological and cross-cultural studies steadily extended our understanding of the factors beyond the individual which influence the pattern of breakdown and recovery. In applying these insights, attempts were made to intervene or alter family or public attitudes. Gradually the concept of community care gained ground and there was an increasing move to treat psychiatric patients without institutionalization in community clinics, in therapeutic social clubs, and in sheltered workshops. Many of those active in milieu therapy were vigorous in this field, and hospital projects were often linked with community and domiciliary plans. An essential part of a rehabilitation programme is the preparation of the family, the home, and the community to receive back the patient long absent in hospital. Any open-door programme involves a programme of public education. Every administrative therapist becomes involved in these activities and must spend time and thought on them. This is, however, not the direct concern of this book, which is examining the doctor's task in treating patients *within* a psychiatric institution. Community and family and social psychiatry will only therefore be discussed where they directly impinge on the work within the hospital.

CHAPTER 3

Therapeutic Milieux

Administrative therapy is the task of constructing a therapeutic milieu for the patients in a psychiatric institution. If we knew what aspects of a milieu, an atmosphere, a way of life, were therapeutic and helpful to patients it might not be too difficult to provide them – though even then we should have to contend with the fallibility of staff (and ourselves) in building and maintaining them. But unfortunately we lack any clear prescription for a therapeutic milieu. We know, from what the social scientists have told us, how antitherapeutic the traditional custodial mental hospital milieu was. There have been a number of exciting experiments and we can see certain fruitful directions, enough to change our own way of functioning markedly. But we have no clear, detailed, unequivocal prescription, and in Chapter 8 some of the reasons for this are examined and possible directions explored.

In the meantime, however, we must act with what we have. It seems therefore valuable to set out some of the principles for organizing the patients' life which are accepted at the present time. Some of these are fully accepted, certain, and proven over the years; others are tentative and controversial. Some of them will be discarded in due course and others will

31

be reformulated. It will be clear, too, that some of them may conflict at times with others. This is inevitable. Correct choice between desirable but incompatible courses of action is an essential part of all administration and of administrative therapy.

BASIC PRINCIPLES

First, then, are the principles of asylum management, hammered out over a century and a half of experience. They were known to Lord Shaftesbury, to Dorothea Lynde Dix, and to Albert Deutsch. It should not be necessary to set them out, but to omit them would give an incomplete picture. Even today there are places where these minimum requirements fail, so that milieu therapy cannot begin.

The general principle is the ancient one, *Primum non nocere*; as Florence Nightingale[40] put it, 'It may seem a strange principle to enumerate as the very first requirement in a hospital that it should do the sick no harm.'

1. The patient must receive sufficient support for life

There must be enough food, clothing, warmth. Two centuries of experience show that these may often fail. One of the first targets of pinch-penny administration is the patient's food.

A well-trained physician took a temporary post in a provincial mental hospital during wartime. He found strange haemorrhagic lesions in an old men's ward. Testing found three cases of frank scurvy and many of subscurvy. For years these toothless men had been on 'soft diet' – mashes of various kinds, all well boiled and devoid of Vitamin C. Fruit had been removed from the hospital diet by the lay administrator on grounds of economy in wartime. The only reason that scurvy was not widespread was because a number of patients had visitors who brought them fruit.

2. The patient must receive adequate medical care and protection from disease

Helpless people do not complain; medical checks by competent doctors are necessary. If a hospital has very few doctors, their entire time may be absorbed in this essential task. This is the case in some state hospitals in the United States. Even in Britain, where the standard of medical staffing and physical care in mental hospitals is fairly high, the physical care of the large frail population takes a great deal of medical time and must at times take priority over psychiatric therapy.

Infectious disease is a danger in any place where people are living closely together. In the asylum days many patients died of infections they acquired within the institution – dysentery, typhoid, tuberculosis – and constant vigilance was needed to find and halt these diseases. Some of the most dehumanizing asylum rituals started as rational precautions against dangerous disease. Though the diseases are less of a threat nowadays and are more easily checked, the dangers may still be present.

A traditional hospital was reviewing the daily life of the long-stay patients in order to eliminate the many humiliating procedures so vividly described by Goffman. Many, such as routine turning out of lockers, counting of cutlery after meals, and communal underwear, were successfully eliminated. Attention fell on the 'bathing parade', when thirty women at a time were herded into a 'general bathroom', stripped naked *en masse*, and scrubbed by sturdy staff members, while their clothing was sorted through.

The scene was phantasmagoric and degrading –the crowds of aged, naked, misshapen grey-headed figures milling about amidst steam, pools of water, and piles of sopping clothing, while the tiled walls re-echoed to shouts, screams, complaints, and splashing.

In a ward of elderly women patients at a good social level, the 'bathing parade' was abolished and they were allowed to bathe individually at their own discretion. They were responsible patients, many years resident, working in hospital departments, mostly diagnosed as paranoid schizophrenics. They expressed gratitude for the change.

Two years later one patient mentioned to a nurse that she was having difficulty in sleeping. The young ward doctor increased her sedation, but after several other patients had made the same complaint he inquired further. They spoke of itching and a rash; he examined them and was puzzled, so requested a visit of a dermatologist, who diagnosed scabies. A survey showed that nearly all the ward were infected.

It took several weeks of treatment and repeated examinations before the infection was stamped out. Investigation showed that one patient had a chronic scabetic condition without any discomfort, that a few of the patients had become more senile and personally neglectful, and that a number had suffered in silence because they did not trust the ward nurse sufficiently to tell her of what they felt was a shameful affliction. After general discussions with staff and patients, a system of bath checks and examinations of less careful patients was worked out.

3. The patient should be protected from abuse and danger
To be given charge of helpless people owning desirable goods is a temptation to a needy person. To be left in charge of

people you believe to be dangerous when you have inadequate training or support tempts a frightened, ignorant person to use illicit violence to maintain control. Recurrent scandals of stealing, beating up, and manslaughter in mental hospitals, even famous ones with 'adequate' and 'well-trained' staff, show that these are real dangers.

A young doctor started training in a famous psychiatric hospital. He was puzzled by a number of curious accidents which befell patients; several suffered fractured ribs and one died of a massive retroperitoneal haemorrhage following a struggle with a staff member. Finally a patient accused a male nurse of punching him. The head nurse was horrified, pointing out that this nurse was a well-trained senior nurse with an excellent Service record. The superintendent held a full investigation, but there were no other witnesses; it was the patient's word against that of the nurse, though the injuries supported the patient's story. The nurse was reprimanded, warned that he was in danger of prosecution, and moved to other work. The incidents ceased. Many months later when they had come to trust him and speak freely, junior nurses told the young doctor more. They said that the senior nurse had told them that he had learned in the Service the necessity of showing violent patients 'who was boss' and had taught the young men how to punch patients so as to hurt and cow them without leaving any traces.

Such incidents are very rare nowadays in British hospitals, but they can still occur, and there have been recent incidents and allegations in American state hospitals.

Any administrator who denies that such things could ever happen in 'his' hospital shows a disturbing ignorance of the difficulties and temptations of some parts of psychiatric nursing and a dangerous blindness to the frailty of human nature. Books are occasionally published with allegations of brutality in mental hospitals. One most valuable book by a former alcoholic patient (Maine[35]) begins with a description of brutalities but then goes on to describe how the author himself became an attendant and came to understand how it was that these things happened. He pointed out that the blame lay not so much with the attendants, untrained, ignorant, and frightened men who were put in charge of wards full of patients whom they could not understand but knew to be violent and left to work out their own methods of control, but with the doctors and the society that put them there and did so little to understand and support them.

One of the advantages of the staff meetings of a therapeutic community is that the staff close beside the patients – the junior nurses, the nursing assistants, the occupational therapist – can share their anxieties, their fears of injury, and their own reactive feelings of aggression with the doctor.

These first three propositions would receive general assent, although some hospitals may fail to implement either the first or the second, and unreflective attempts to prevent abuses have been the root of many antitherapeutic regulations. The next two propositions raise more controversial issues, but are set out to draw attention to the dilemmas that arise.

4. The patient should be protected from the results of his own impulses

It seems reasonable that an institution should not let a hypomanic spend all his money, should not let a melancholic patient kill himself, should not let a confused and fatuous woman become pregnant, should not let an impulsive man add yet another killing to his score. Yet the attempt to guard against these disasters has been the given reason for the multiplication of locks and antisuicidal precautions that finally made mental hospitals custodial places that bred institutionalization. In the custodial hospitals patients railed against the restrictions placed on them and challenged the doctors to justify them. The answer, 'We are doing it for your own good!' rang very hollow. Yet this is at times true.

A recurrent hypomanic businessman was becoming over-active again. His family were beginning to take steps when he went downtown to an auction of paintings; in his elation he overvalued them and ran the bidding up. He was committed the following day but his family found themselves saddled with forty indifferent daubs which had to be resold at considerable loss. In the remorseful period of his recovery he blamed them bitterly for not having had him committed earlier.

5. The needs of the patients should be the first concern of the hospital

As stated this seems an unassailable proposition. Yet in fact they often become a secondary concern. Mental hospitals are often regarded as places of detention and the 'safety of the public' is at times stated to be more important than the needs of the patient. This has always been an area of difficulty and controversy and at times the general community has required the mental hospital to act as a place of custody. The mental hospitals in Britain have since 1948 been part of a hospital service, and, especially since the Mental Health Act 1959, there has been little expectation that they should provide secure custody; there have been some protests from judges who wish for a place of secure custody to which to send people. Some American state hospitals may be required to hold accused persons pending trial, or even to hold convicted persons. In such hospitals much of the energies of the medical and attendant staff are taken up with activities directed against the (antisocial) patient for the benefit of society.

I have stated these generally accepted principles baldly to draw attention to them. It can be said that the general establishment of these was the achievement of a century and a half of organized psychiatry in Britain, from the setting up of the first Metropolitan Commissioners in Lunacy in 1828 following the revelations of the abuses of Bethlem and the private madhouses until the dissolution of the Board of Control in 1960. Unfortunately, this also produced the stultifying, prison-like atmosphere of the older mental hospitals and the widespread institutionalization. Our present task is gently to tip out the bath water of institutionalization without losing the baby of adequate protection of the patients from danger, abuse, and neglect.

MODERN GENERAL PRINCIPLES

These were summarized in the 1953 report of the WHO Expert Committee on Mental Health[59] arising from the experience of Kraus, Rees, and Sivadon. They began by saying that the 'atmosphere' of the hospital was 'the most important single factor in the efficacy of the treatment given'.

They then discussed constituents of this atmosphere.

1. Preservation of the Patient's Personality

'In too many psychiatric hospitals still the patient is robbed of her personal possessions, her clothes, her name and should her head be lousy, even her hair. Every step, therefore, that can encourage the patient's self-respect and sense of identity should be taken even at the cost of considerable inconvenience.'

The schizophrenic is disorganized and confused; the melancholic feels worthless and degraded; nearly all persons entering mental hospitals voluntarily or under compulsion feel discarded, unwanted, and rejected by society. It is essential that these feelings should not be compounded by the institution; every attempt must be made to retain anything which stresses their identity and links with the outside world. But this does mean considerable inconvenience; it is easier and cheaper to administer an institution where everyone has identical personal possessions – and as few as possible. This eases laundering, reduces accounting, and discourages thieving. The tidy-minded bureaucrats will always move towards it. Goffman has suggested that there may be a deeper need for those in total institutions to strip an entrant of those things that remind him of his previous identity outside; he points to monasteries and nunneries where entrants enthusiastically submit to all the indignities listed above, abandoning all personal goods, cutting off their hair, putting on a habit designed to be shapeless. The attempt to preserve the patient's sense of individuality, so important for recovery, is a constant fight against social pressures and 'administrative' arguments. The need for individual considerations is always liable to be in conflict with the needs of the mass; this dilemma becomes worse as the size of the institution increases.

2. *Trust the Patients*
The WHO Committee writes:

> 'Another element in this atmosphere is *the assumption that patients are trustworthy* until their behaviour proves

the contrary to be true. The locking of wards creates the urge to escape; the removal of knives and other elaborate and insulting precautions have provoked many suicidal attempts. High walls, bars, armour-plated windows, bunches of keys, uniform clothing, and all the other paraphernalia of the prison make modern psychiatric treatment impossible. It has now been amply demonstrated that only a very small minority of patients needs to be in locked wards in a well-run mental hospital.

'Patients must not only be assumed to be trustworthy; they must also be assumed to retain *the capacity for a considerable degree of responsibility and initiative*. The running of many activities, therefore, in the therapeutic community which the modern psychiatric hospital should be, should devolve upon the patients themselves.'

This has not proved too difficult to maintain once a basic shift in orientation of the whole hospital has been achieved. So long as the emphasis of the institution is on prevention and custody, then everyone will constantly emphasize the untrustworthiness of those directly below them and spend most of their time checking up and penalizing. Once a general policy of promoting personal growth of both patients and staff has been generally established, all except the very authoritarian personalities will find occasion for extending trust and opportunity to those under them.

3. Activity and Work

'*Activity*, in fact, is one of the most important characteristics of the therapeutic community. But it should be planned and purposeful activity, and the planning of the patient's day is probably the most important therapeutic task of the hospital psychiatrist.'

As the historical chapter indicated, the organization of a day of meaningful work has been a cornerstone of every therapeutic milieu from Pinel to Maxwell Jones. There have been many types of activity, all with different rationales. Much purposeless idleness is one of the striking and constant characteristics of poor mental hospitals. Organizing of work calls for diligence and persistence by the therapists. The WHO authors make a number of suggestions about the need for graduated work and responsibility. Considerable ingenuity is needed to find meaningful work for impaired persons, and the bigger the hospital and the more its departments are modernized, the more difficult this becomes. There have been many arguments whether work should be 'creative' or 'repetitive'; whether it should be paid or not; whether it should be industrial or agricultural. We are only beginning to establish some scientific findings about the kinds of incentive that operate effectively in work therapy.

4. Staff Attitudes and Relationships
The Committee had some comments on this:

> 'As in the community at large, one of the most characteristic aspects of the psychiatric hospital is the type of relationship between people that are to be found within it. The nature of the relationships between the medical director and his staff will be reflected in the relationship between the psychiatric staff and the nurses, and finally in the relationship not only between the nurses and the patients, but between the patients themselves. . . .
>
> 'The creation of the milieu of a therapeutic community and the fostering of the relationships and activities which compose it are the therapeutic task of the medical director.'

41

5. Sanctions

The Committee discussed aberrant behaviour.

'This does not imply that disturbing behaviour on the part of a patient should be ignored. On the contrary, *good behaviour* must be encouraged and antisocial behaviour met by appropriate measures. The patient who disturbs others must be removed and told why – not as a punishment, but because he disturbs others – but he should be reintroduced at the earliest opportunity.'

These proposals in themselves are sound, but they do not begin to consider the mass of tangled and frightening feelings that staff and other patients have towards disturbing behaviour, and the WHO Committee did not fully consider the vital question of the checking of undesirable activities of patients and staff. The nineteenth-century approach of control by laws, fault-finding inquiries, and punishment, though it checked gross abuses, produced the custodial asylums and institutionalization. Only with the therapeutic-community concept of peer-group control have we begun to open the possibility of a way of checking deviant behaviour that does not bind the whole institution in paralysing penal rules.

PRINCIPLES OF THE THERAPEUTIC COMMUNITY

The excellent and striking phrase 'therapeutic community' coined by Main in 1946 has now had so much currency that it has been almost rubbed smooth of meaning. At times it seems that its use means nothing more than that someone knows the up-to-date and modish phrase. Apart from misuse, the term has, however, been applied to two different 'communities'; to a whole hospital of many hundreds of people, or to a small unit where face-to-face relationships between all staff and patients are possible (such as a ward, or a group of wards). The WHO Committee[59] used the word in the first sense when they said the psychiatric hospital had to play the role of a therapeutic community. In more recent times the phrase has been mostly restricted to the smaller units and will be used in this sense here.

Maxwell Jones,[30] who has given the word meaning, stated that he described 'a therapeutic community as distinctive among other comparable treatment centres in the way the institution's total resources, both staff and patients, are self-consciously pooled in furthering treatment'. Martin[37] said that a therapeutic community is one 'in which a deliberate effort is made to use to the fullest possible extent in a comprehensive treatment plan the contributions of all staff and patients'.

These two statements set forth the common and new principle of the therapeutic-community idea – of deliberately using the contributions of *all* – especially the less highly trained staff and the other patients – in the attempt to help the sick individual. In the traditional psychiatric hospital many patients received help from other patients or from aides and junior staff. In autobiographies ex-patients often mention how some act of kindness or gesture of understanding from someone close by first penetrated the fog of fear, suspicion, and confusion. Yet such actions were often unofficial and sometimes even against regulations. Some of the advice given by attendants or other patients, however, must at times have been unhelpful, for they lacked knowledge of all of an individual's circumstances. The therapeutic community is an attempt to harness these forces and use them helpfully.

Maxwell Jones began his first therapeutic community in 1940. Since that time there have been many, and many descriptions of them. The method has been applied to psychopathic personalities, to persons with psychoneuroses and with psychoses, to groups of patients in individual analysis, to prisoners, and to others.

Despite all the descriptions, there have been few clear statements of the essential characteristics of a therapeutic community. Denber[19] summarizing a 1959 Conference reported that forty-five experts discussed the therapeutic community for three days but that 'an exact definition of this concept was not attempted'. Maxwell Jones himself has never laid down rigid criteria of what constitutes a therapeutic community, and rigidity would be out of place in a developing concept. He says:

'The fact is, of course, that there is, as yet, no one model of a therapeutic community and all that is intended is that it should mobilize the interest, skills and enthusiasms of staff and patients and give them sufficient freedom of action to create their own optimal treatment and living conditions. Under such circumstances, what will emerge will be characteristic for the particular group and may have little in common with other therapeutic communities. My own feeling is that doctors should not slavishly copy a particular model but simply work in a way which is most compatible for all the staff concerned' [30] (p. 73).

However, certain characteristics can be stated which have been seen in most therapeutic communities.

1. Freeing of Communications

A constant effort is made to open communications and to free the many blocks that exist, both between individuals and between different status levels within the community. This gives the senior staff some chance to know of significant emotional happenings directly from those involved; it lets patients and junior staff know what senior medical or nursing policy is. This of course is an endless process; new blockages of information and collusions are forever developing and must be loosened and examined in their turn.

2. Analysis of all Events in the therapeutic community in terms of individual and interpersonal dynamics. This is practised at all times, but particularly in the meetings; every happening is relevant and everyone may be able to gain something of value from understanding it better. This, of course, presupposes an acceptance of some psychodynamic theory of interpersonal relations, though this is fairly general in our culture nowadays. Many situations, however, can be quite usefully analysed in terms of observed happenings and admitted feelings without too many interpretive postulations of unconscious urges and the inevitable denials these arouse.

3. Provision of Learning Experiences
Apart from those occurring spontaneously, there is a deliberate attempt in workshops, outings, dances, etc., to provide quasi-natural settings in which methods of personal functioning may be changed and new patterns tried out.

4. Flattening of the Authority Pyramid
Opening communications eliminates many of the hierarchical layers which so blocked the workings of the traditional ward. There is, for instance, direct contact between psychiatrist and attendant, or patient and staff nurse. This means that patients and junior staff feel more free to make comments or propose actions instead of refraining for fear they may get into trouble. The flattening, however, threatens many

professionally inculcated attitudes and personal securities particularly in the middle-status members of the hierarchy, such as charge nurses and junior doctors.

5. Role-Examination

At differing times all members of the community are called on to examine what they are doing, why, and how it affects others. This helps the patients to modify their behaviour towards other people and the staff to modify their way of working. With this often goes some role-blurring so that people become able to do parts of the task of others.

6. Community Meeting

This is the main forum for most of these processes and is often considered the main characteristic of the therapeutic community. Regularly, preferably daily, all members of the community assemble, usually for an hour. All matters of general concern are discussed. The general pattern is of great informality; anyone is free to speak, and the less direction by the nurse or the doctor, the better. Emotional interactions are valuable, though therapeutic communities containing violent people have found aggression should remain verbal and that open violence is seldom therapeutically valuable. A staff meeting follows the community meeting. This is essential to allow the staff to work through the material and their own aroused feelings and also to work out policy problems.

Other group meetings, large and small, are commonly organized round work projects, outings, staff seminars, etc. They will vary in formality and in task orientation but all of them are opportunities for interaction and trying out of roles.

CHAPTER 4

Administrative Therapy

We can now examine the practice of administrative therapy – the physician's task in the psychiatric institution.

The work of the social scientists taught us much about what happened in our hospitals, forced us to realize the social factors affecting the person who spends a long time in an institution, and suggested the possibility of milieu therapy – of harnessing some of those forces. The experiments of the last two decades have empirically established certain principles which seem important in creating a social system in which impaired individuals will move toward greater independence and effectiveness. The descriptions of therapeutic communities, in particular the writings of Maxwell Jones, Rapoport, Wilmer, and Martin, give a general picture of this social system. What is the particular contribution of the doctor?

This book is explicitly designed for physicians, and what follows is seen from the doctor's viewpoint. The roles of other people in the therapeutic community change considerably and for some of them, especially the trained psychiatric nurse, the changes are as painful and as rewarding as those necessary for the doctors. But these have been discussed by other writers, so the reference to them will be incidental.

Administrative Therapy

Before treatment comes diagnosis; before diagnosis, examination. Following these time-honoured medical principles, the administrative therapist must examine, must assess, his institution. The full assessment of an institution and its social system is the task of a sociologist, but the doctor can acquire some competence, and will need it if he is to plan his actions usefully.

ASSESSMENT

What can be done depends on what you have got. The possibilities of administrative therapy in any situation depend on the institution – its size, function, traditions, and facilities; on the patients – their numbers, the types of illnesses, the way they are selected to enter and their length of stay; on the staff – their degree of training, their professional groupings, their previous experience; and not least on the administrative therapist himself – his status in the institution, his skill, knowledge, and experience.

An assessment of the institution or unit is a useful and necessary exercise. It will clarify issues and, in doing so, indicate possibilities and limitations. The assessment can be compared to the clinical interview that precedes psychotherapeutic treatment; during this interview the condition of the patient is assessed, his problems and his potentialities reviewed, and the possible methods of treatment considered. Of an institution, one asks: What is the function of this unit? What task has it been given by society? What sort of patient is sent here? What sort of results are to be achieved? An analysis of the functions of a psychiatric institution may reveal anomalies and inconsistencies, and even incompatible functions such as its use by society both as a hospital for treatment and as a prison for punishment. These very often limit its development. One can also ask how efficiently the unit carries out the function given it by society; the failings will indicate areas for study.

About a year after becoming medical superintendent of Fulbourn Hospital I was asked by the local voluntary Mental Welfare Association to address them on a subject of my choice. I chose to speak on the subject that was interesting and puzzling me most at that time and the talk was subsequently published as 'Functions of the Mental Hospital'.[15] This is now in many ways out of date. But it does represent an attempt at assessment of a task of administrative therapy. In particular it discusses the tasks that English society in the mid 1950s set a psychiatric hospital, showed how some conflicted with others and indicated how we might approach them.

The general demands of society will set limits and possibilities. So also will the special circumstances of the unit and its framework of finance, government, and responsibility. The director of a private sanatorium has considerable freedom in spending money and varying treatment patterns but must ensure that there are enough fees coming in to meet the expenses. A state hospital director can accept any patient, but is under constant pressure to economize on public funds and is open to criticism from elected representatives if social experiments are so bold as to shock the righteous. Within the British National Health Service some mental hospitals have their own Management Committees, which gives a chance of a policy sensitive to the needs of the psychiatric patients, but many are grouped with non-psychiatric institutions and may find their special needs misunderstood. When the unit is one within a hospital, the policies and attitudes of senior staff may be very important. A head nurse or medical superintendent who is unsympathetic or though sympathetic is timorous and easily frightened by agitation, will limit greatly the amount of social restructuring that can be done or the speed at which it can go. For the ward doctor the attitude of his medical superiors will be very important. In the writings about therapeutic communities the expressions of indebtedness to seniors at the end of the articles have often been not the usual pious platitudes but heartfelt thanks for sturdy support through storms and tribulations.

All these external factors, social, governmental, and personal must be assessed. The internal assets must next be considered. What sort of people are there, as patients and as staff? What are their prospects of change? What degree of intelligence, training, and experience do the staff have? What is the social and the economic background of the patients? The developments possible in a small private hospital with upper-middle-class patients and staffed by qualified nurses, are quite different from those in a state hospital ward with labouring-class patients and staff who have had little formal training at all. It should not be thought that the advantages are all with the former; some training can so limit an individual's spontaneity that she is incapable of employing her personality in an effective therapeutic manner.

Apart from the functions and assets of the unit, its social characteristics can also be assessed, in particular the communications network and the authority structure. Fine details of the informal structure will only be learned over the years but gross details can be seen early and may again indicate possibilities or set limitations. Who are the dominant personalities? How do they get on with one another? When are they going to retire? Who is related to whom? (In many mental hospitals there is a network of staff intermarriages of great importance in the informal structure of the institution.) It is important also to identify the culture-carriers of the community. This anthropological term means those members of a society who transmit (and embody) the values and traditions of the culture; they are the people who give guidance, who know what was done before and what should be done now, who see themselves as committed members of the society and value its traditions. They are not so much the leaders as the established, respected members of standing.

In any society there are a number of culture-carriers. It is their beliefs that govern what is done, and unless they change their views, all reform will be transient. In a traditional psychiatric hospital, as Belknap[6] has pointed out, they are the senior charge nurses and attendants; in a long-stay ward they are usually certain of the working patients, often the ward domestics, and, occasionally, nursing assistants.

There are different ways of carrying out the assessment. Where the doctor is already in post, and the unit is considering changing its function, he can work from his own knowledge. His difficulty is that he will take things for granted and not question long-accepted practices. Anthropologists say that you can study any society but your own. It is difficult for a doctor to think freshly about his own hospital. He can enlarge his picture by talking with his staff and patients, if they are ready for this. The device of employing an external agent, a social scientist, or a questionnaire team creates problems of their introduction, of the anxieties aroused by their questions and the disappointments if these are not acted upon, and they may well cause more problems than they solve.

The medical superintendent of a liberal and well-known English mental hospital and his senior medical colleagues felt that it would be valuable to know something of staff attitudes. They obtained a grant for a study from a national foundation and permission from the Hospital Management Committee. A national body specializing in such surveys was employed. They came and spent many months at the hospital holding confidential interviews with all grades of staff. The staff nurses (especially the men) were very hesitant and asked what would be done with the opinions recorded; after reassurance they agreed to co-operate. The report finally returned. The analysis reported good morale, but inevitably detailed many dissatisfactions. The report so upset the Hospital Management Committee that they said it must not be made public. Then the staff began to ask what had happened to the material, so a brief report was issued to them; they soon knew, however, that it was a censored, watered-down version. In talking of it afterwards, everyone regretted the exercise. The medical superintendent said that though the survey had revealed a few unrecognized problems that were easily righted, it had caused far too much upset. The nursing staff were left unhappy and suspicious. Years later, in another hospital, a man who had been a staff nurse at the time of the questionnaire was unwilling to co-operate with another inquiry, saying that they collected confidential opinions, that no one knew where they went, and that they were bad for the whole hospital.

With a new doctor coming in, the problem is more complex. He has the advantage of being new to the institution, so that he can see its characteristics clearly, and depending on his experience, can assess the unit well. On the other hand, he faces all sorts of social pressures because he is the 'new man' coming in. His arrival will have been preceded by rumours and during his early days all his behaviour is being watched by hundreds of eyes. Is he tough? Is he odd? What does he like? What does he dislike? Many anxious people will be attempting to manoeuvre him into supporting their positions. There is a temptation on him to 'institute reforms' right away; to come in with ready-made solutions and insist on their immediate implementation. Though this may possibly be successful behaviour in a business tycoon, and can be a method of administration, it is not administrative therapy. It does not help the staff toward maturity or independence, and recreates the old authoritarian hierarchy. Though there may be immediate benefits for the patients, especially in physical comforts, it is unlikely that this will provide them, in the end, with the atmosphere of encouragement toward independence and spontaneity that they require. The incoming doctor would do better to fit into the role assigned to him, do what is expected of him, and listen and think. People will try him out – and reveal themselves. They will tell him the burning problems of the unit; these he can make his first priority. It is almost certainly unwise to rush into a unit with a preconceived plan to be forced through despite all opposition. Though the plan may succeed, a pattern has been established of problem solving by administrative fiat, by *Führer-prinzip*, and the development of problem solving by the staff inhibited.

ACTION

Communications

A first step in modifying the social structure of a community to a more therapeutic pattern is to open new communications. This can often best be done by means of group meetings and group problem-solving. Some important problem will soon present itself; instead of imposing a solution, the doctor can call the people involved together and let them talk about it. They may never have met in this particular grouping before. Even if they have, under the pressure of the problem there will be mutual exploration and clarification of attitudes, and skilfully led, they will work toward a solution. As they achieve one, they will see the advantages of group problem-solving. (It is wise, for the first few meetings, to choose a problem that it is within the power of the group to solve.) In these meetings all happenings can be analysed in the presence of all involved and newer and better ways of functioning worked out. Care must be taken, however, to prepare adequately. When the upper members of any authority-pyramid communicate with the lower ranks, they threaten those in the middle. When the doctor speaks to the patients or to the student nurses, he threatens the charge nurses. When the charge attendant speaks to the patients, he threatens the junior members of the staff. When the consultant psychiatrist talks with the nurses, he threatens the nursing administrators and the junior doctors. These anxieties are natural and inevitable and steps should be taken to meet them and to support the middle-rank members until they begin to see that they too have a good deal to gain from change. The opening of communications is a slow process and will develop only gradually. It is also a painful one. The doctor himself will be made aware of the severity of problems that he had not previously appreciated and from which he had been insulated by the traditional communications structure of the psychiatric hospital.

As communications open up, it will become possible to modify the authority structure and to allow junior members of the staff to take more responsible roles; the decision, for instance, about who shall have permission to leave the ward can gradually be transferred down, first from the doctors to the nurses, then to the ward meeting, and finally may even be decided by the patients themselves. In all this the aim is to enable the patients to grow and to exercise as much responsible authority as they can for their own lives as a preparation for ultimately leaving the unit.

The administrative therapist should try to draw in every person's contribution, and can ask himself, 'Is there anyone whose views we have not heard?' At an administrative level, this may be the catering officer or the storeman; among the ward staff it may be the kitchen maid or the key patient worker; at the ward meeting it may be the delinquent member being discussed while he is absent. Discussion can be postponed until the absentee attends and a solution gradually worked out. In these ways the doctor can demonstrate those general principles of community decision-making that promote personality growth in the patients or the staff members concerned; namely, respect for the needs and attitudes of the individual, a sympathetic hearing for all, statement of the needs of the group, and an appreciation of the realities of the situation, combining to work out an effective plan which is then carried through.

Authority

An examination of the authority structure of the unit nearly always reveals the need for modification. In the traditional psychiatric institution there is tremendous centralization of decision-making, with the inevitable erection (because of the numbers involved) of a hierarchical pyramid of authority. In the ward, all sorts of matters are brought to the doctor for his decision; he has to sign for medical treatment and for drugs; he has to sign paroles and passes; he has to answer all letters; he often has to sign for any scarce article such as orange juice or toilet soap. At the hospital level the process can go even further; all letters must be signed by the medical superintendent; all repainting schemes must be decided by the medical superintendent; all patients for discharge (even when there are scores each week) must be seen by the medical superintendent, and so on. The doctor is constantly making decisions for which he lacks the time or the necessary knowledge; worse, other capable people – junior doctors, nurses, attendants, sensible patients – are handed down orders which seem foolish in the light of their (better) knowledge of the situation.

This bizarre situation is the end-result of two themes of the traditional psychiatric institution: the medical model by which the doctor alone can make decisions about the patient, and the century-old tradition of fault-finding authority. Boards of Control, Committees of Visitors, Congressional investigations, sought someone to blame for mishaps and errors, so they laid the blame on the man at the top and insisted that he be responsible. Ultimately this can produce an institution that is a caricature of a governmental bureaucracy rather than a hospital, where everyone will pass information upward rather than take a decision, where each person is fearful of the tyranny of those above him and convinced of the incompetence, ignorance, and wickedness of those below him. The result is that either no decision or a wrongly informed decision is made; this may avoid lawsuits, but is bad for the patients.

The doctor can start modifying this immediately, by querying why things are brought to him for decision and by delegating all decisions that he can. He will find that nurses and others will be willing to take decisions, once he makes it clear that he will back them. The difficulty, of course, comes when something goes wrong; this is a major test of the administrative therapist. If he says, 'Well, next time ask *me*!' he is reinstating the old authority structure. This is the critical

56

situation with all delegated authority and is well understood by anyone who has held power in a human organization, be it a factory, army, or business office, but it may be new to a doctor reared in the medical model of retaining personal responsibility for decision. He will learn to support the nurse's growing independence, while helping her to function better on the next occasion.

The aim of all this change is to make the person next to the patient capable of making the most helpful and growth-promoting decision. The point at which milieu therapy takes effect is with the patient when he does something – when he refuses, or accepts, food, or when he makes an advance or a withdrawal, when he grasps a hand extended to him, or bites it. What comes next depends on the state of mind of the person there—usually an attendant or another patient – and this depends on how free he feels to do what he senses is right, how much he knows about the patient, what models for behaviour he has been given.

A woman patient on a 'disturbed ward' made strangling attacks on staff. The ward was organized on traditional lines; the standing instructions were – if there is a struggle call for other staff; if you cannot quieten the patient give the 'S.O.S' sedation or call the medical officer who will give an injection. This did not control the situation. The attacks increased and the patient became the main 'problem case'. A senior nurse was injured; nurses began to request transfers or to stay off duty with minor complaints; a woman doctor requested instruction in jujitsu. The patient denied all knowledge of the attacks and remained confused, hostile, bitter, and uncommunicative during interviews with the doctors; attempts at psychotherapy made no progress. She was frequently secluded; more sedation had to be given; intensive ECT was used for a time; a leucotomy was discussed.

The attacks continued into the period when the ward was being restructured towards a therapeutic community. The attacks were discussed at the staff meetings. It emerged in the staff discussions that she 'went glassy-eyed' before attacking someone and this was linked with the fact that she had been a medium. The consultant psychiatrist explained the mechanisms of hysterical dissociation and trances to the staff group. The social worker reminded the group that the patient had been admitted following an attempt to kill her husband's mistress. As the discussion proceeded from week to week, the demands for medical action became fewer, and proposals came forward. A nursing assistant reported that a damp cloth on the forehead sometimes brought the patient round; the occupational therapist reported that if she reminded the patient who she was and emphasized that she was not the hated paramour, the attack ceased. Other staff reported success in dealing with the episodes, and also attempts to occupy the patient in other ways. The staff anxiety about the attacks decreased and they were reported unemotionally. Ward meetings started about this time and several 'strangling episodes' occurred during these, especially towards the social worker who was seeing the husband. After a few moments the trance passed and the patient wept bitterly when the other patients told her what they had witnessed; by now they, who had been very frightened by the attacks, all knew of the home situation. Gradually the attacks declined until six months later no more were occurring, and the patient was discussing freely her feelings about her supplanter and making realistic plans to leave hospital and take up life on her own. She had also deployed her considerable talents in organizing activities and dances within the ward.

The doctors here had failed while they continued traditional medical treatment, but succeeded when they concentrated on assisting those in direct contact with the patient.

At the hospital level there is great need to examine the authority structure. British mental hospitals have been bedevilled for a decade by tussles between insecure medical superintendents and thrusting consultant psychiatrists about who should make decisions – sign letters, see relatives, admit patients, discharge patients, etc. The Mental Health Act 1959 removed the legal basis for interference, though there are still residual grievances. Just removing the tyranny of the medical superintendent is not enough. An honest examination of the authority structure is needed. If freedom is good for consultant psychiatrists it is good for those working under them too, and there is a danger that the successful leader of revolt will himself become a petty tyrant. Consultant psychiatrists in examining their operations have found themselves using the same arguments based on legal responsibility to their juniors that the medical superintendents used against them, thus still keeping everyone, but finally the patient, resentfully dependent.

Role-Alteration

Changing the social structure changes people's tasks. Some have more to do, some less. Most people will comment on a change in their work and some will protest. One of the main tasks of staff meetings is to analyse and expedite these changes. The task of the administrative therapist is to understand that this will occur and to ease the change. Typically this stress falls on the registered nurse when aides take part in therapy, on the senior charge nurse when young nurses start taking initiative, on doctors when social workers display greater psychodynamic sophistication, on social workers when attendants show an ability to handle relatives better. The administrative therapist should know who will be feeling the pinch of change and help them with this; talk to them personally beforehand, let them ventilate their anxieties while he assures them of his continuing regard and support, help them to talk about this in staff meetings. Gradually differing members of the therapeutic team will come to understand others' work better; they will take over portions of it, and give up some of their own functions. There will be a tendency to 'role-blurring', that is, tasks will be performed by any member of the staff team regardless of previous training. This is inevitable but there is no evidence that it is in itself valuable. There is a tendency for every staff member to be a 'jack of all trades but master of none' and there is a drift toward abdication of professional responsibility which is tempting to some doctors who find the making of unpopular or grave decisions painful. Role-change is inevitable, and role-redefinition desirable, but any role-blurring should be carefully examined and its value to the patient's treatment critically assessed.

A therapeutic community had been developing enthusiastically in an admitting unit. The question of permission for weekend leave had been raised and discussed and the staff had transferred this problem to the patients, who decided by vote who should go out. The medical director came to feel that these decisions were being taken too lightly and that weekend leave was being granted to people whom he did not consider suitable. In discussions with colleagues he came to realize that he had confused informed opinion with responsibility. The patients knew one another's behaviour and had a very good idea who was fit for leave; he was, however, the medical director and he would personally be held responsible if a patient from the unit committed suicide, violence, or crime when on weekend leave. He put this to the staff and then to the patients, all of whom saw the point. The system was changed; the patients considered applications for leave at their meetings; those that they recommended went to the medical director who granted them if he felt he could trust the individual. Thus the patients' informed observations were obtained, but the responsibility remained with the man to whom outside society had given it.

MEDICAL ROLE-CHANGE

The doctor who starts administrative therapy is stepping out of his traditional medical role. He is taking part in the running of the unit. Later the effects of this on him and his self-image will be fully discussed; but some effects must be mentioned now.

As a doctor becomes an administrative therapist his own self-image will change; he will learn to see himself not as the omnipotent medical expert (an image fostered by the general teaching hospitals, in surgical firms and other situations) but as a member of a team, a member with high skills, but nevertheless just a member. He will learn to think in terms of 'we' not 'I' and learn a certain amount of humility. This sounds reasonable, but is in fact difficult for most doctors. Doctors have been trained to take decisions and carry the responsibility for them personally. They have learned to think of nurses, social workers, and occupational therapists as being 'under medical direction'. This is true of certain matters traditionally set aside for the doctor. But when he takes the chair in a discussion of how a particular patient is to be nursed or occupied, or how the kitchen staff can get the patients' meals out quicker to the wards, these are their expert fields and his may be no better than a lay opinion. The doctor has to learn to be a team member, albeit an important one; to accept the team decisions and work with them. Patterson[43] has discussed the difference between 'sapiential' authority – that granted to a man because of his knowledge and skill, and 'structural' authority – that given a man because of his position. He pointed out that doctors in charge of mental hospitals, or hospital wards, are particularly likely to confuse these; that they often are acting as members of an administrative or therapeutic team rather than as medical experts, and on such matters as carpets or pig-rearing their opinion is not necessarily better than that of any other person present.

As the therapeutic community develops, the medical role-change will extend and the doctor will find more happening to him. At first he will meet respectful discussion of his proposals. Then there will be disagreement. Then, in due course, there will be comment on the way he is doing his job. It is a tremendous advance for a group of nurses to tell a doctor that they do not think he handled a certain problem well, or that there are certain things that are their job, not his. Much future advance will depend on whether he can accept these comments positively, and not resent criticism. In any criticism of any senior authority there is a component of unresolved Oedipal feeling in the criticizer. It is easy for a psychiatrist to see this; with an analytic patient it is his duty to point it out; with a colleague it is his duty to refrain from what will be regarded as a cheap psycho-analytic trick for crushing fair comment. The onlookers are usually the best judges of the truth of the comment. For the administrative therapist himself, when smarting from a shrewd dig, the best yardstick is probably its relevance to the common task.

Finally a degree of sophistication may be reached where honest personal analysis and interpretation may be acceptable. Doctors are free with their interpretations of the unconscious roots of patients' behaviour. In the open society of the therapeutic community there will come times when the irrational component of anyone's behaviour will be apparent, including that of the doctor himself. It is a measure of his maturity and the security of the group if they can offer an interpretative comment and he can accept it.

LEADERSHIP TASKS IN THE THERAPEUTIC COMMUNITY

The word 'leader' has gradually acquired certain unfortunate connotations, but no better word has yet been forthcoming to describe that member of a group to whom certain tasks necessary to the group's existence are given. We shall here mention some leadership tasks that appear important in the therapeutic milieu. These need not all be taken by the doctor; some of them, at times, will be performed by others. But he may have to undertake any of them.

Group Conductor

Someone must act as conductor, or chairman, of groups and particularly of the community meeting, if only to indicate the beginning and end of the meeting. In the early days this is a most important task, as a pattern of discussing, of behaving and proceeding will be set. It is of great value for an initiator to have had previous experience. Group analytic psychotherapy is the best preparation for conducting a ward community meeting; ordinary committee chairmanship is useful preparation for a medical superintendent. Acting as a committee chairman or conducting a therapeutic group are both learned skills. In each there is a component of technical knowledge – in chairmanship, the rules of procedure, the proper ways to take an agenda, to control discussion, to take motions and amendments and counter-amendments; in group therapy, knowledge of how to select patients, to introduce them, how to direct the floating discussion, to handle silences or to terminate attendance. In both situations there is a far greater component of skill and emotional learning. Each man learns what he can do with his personality and then gradually improves his performance.

The conductor of a meeting will learn in particular to control and assess his own anxiety, and to base his contributions on the needs of the group rather than on his own uneasiness. The ability to refrain from comment, to let other people give the answer, to allow the tension to mount, often comes first. Passivity and abdication are also faults to which some are prone and the conductor fails his group if he cannot at times take action.

The possible range of personality deployment varies. There are excellent administrative therapists who are mostly passive and silent, others who are ebullient, talkative, and aggressive, others vigorous and constantly pressing toward action. Each administrative therapist – like every psychotherapist – must work out his own style and then learn which situations it fits and when it does not do so well.

Group Interpreter

This function is often part of conducting but can also be split off from it. In the well-developed therapeutic community this leadership task is well distributed; patients and staff members make valuable interpretations. Very often interpretations come better from someone who is watching what is happening than from the conductor, who is concerned with the tensions and movements of feeling within the meeting. In the early days of the group, however, the psychiatrist, as the man with psychotherapeutic experience and knowledge of the books of psychopathology, will tend to be the model. Whatever mode of interpretation is finally established – group-centred, individual-centred, 'Freudian', 'Adlerian', 'here-and-now', jargon bespattered, or plainly descriptive – will be an amalgam of the styles and knowledge of the more respected members of the team, of whom the senior psychiatrist is the most influential.

Goal-Setting and Slogan-Choosing

A ward or hospital community is a living concern, frequently undertaking tasks. These are very important for its health. In a work project, people are bound together; they form new relationships and find new roles for themselves. It is important that the community undertakes projects that it can accomplish. To start on a group project and fail is disheartening. The senior members of the ward or the hospital, doctors, nurses, and others, can best judge what is possible and have an important and delicate task choosing between the projects thrown up. Shoenberg[48] in her accounts of the Goodmayes Unit made a point of the necessity to choose goals for that group of schizophrenic patients which were attainable in a reasonably short time.

Slogans are also important. Sometimes the doctor may have the talent to choose them himself; more often they will emerge. But the leaders of the group have much to do with choosing them, for once they emerge they become the focus of loyalties, fears, and hostilities. 'Open doors' has been a most valuable rallying cry for many hospitals.

Spokesman

Someone must speak for the unit in its relations with other bodies. Sometimes it will be the task of the head nurse of the ward to battle with the director of nursing; sometimes a patient will approach an outside group. But usually this task falls to the doctor, because he has the professional status, and outside bodies expect a doctor to speak for a medical unit.

The group will expect the doctor to speak for them and be their representative and spokesman in areas outside of the community, to stand up for them, to fight their battles, to get them necessary supplies, to ward off attacks, or to prevent them being closed down. The ward doctor will be expected to explain the needs of the ward to the matron, the chief male nurse, the medical superintendent, the group secretary, and the hospital management committee. The director of a therapeutic community will be expected to explain their needs to the larger hospital, as Maxwell Jones explained the needs of the Unit to the Belmont Hospital Management Committee and as Wilmer explained the needs of the Oakland Unit to the Admirals who were ultimately responsible.

Many of the great administrative therapists embarked on this task with a happy fury that endeared them greatly to those for whom they were battling. Pinel faced the Revolutionary Tribunal, Conolly battled endlessly with his Committee of Visitors, Maxwell Jones was untiring in defending his unit against Subcommittees of Inquiry from above. Linked with this is the judicious management of external hostility. Nothing unites a group like a common enemy; often a common enemy will help a therapeutic community over a disintegrative phase until they have a chance to carry on with the therapeutic task of analysis. Any institution containing psychiatric patients is the recipient of some stigma

66

and hostility from outside society. It is a matter of judgement
when to ignore and when to stress this.

FLEXIBILITY OF AUTHORITY

One of the major themes of therapeutic communities has
been the retreat from authoritarian attitudes and the development of permissiveness. This has, however, at times
developed into a distaste for any firm action in any circumstances. Rapoport[44] analysed this in his Belmont study and he
observed that occasionally the doctors were forced to have a
patient removed by a duly authorized officer to a mental
hospital, or by the police to jail, and that they felt very guilty
about this. He pointed out that they had been performing a
necessary leadership function; that the community was
threatened with disintegration and that they had to take firm
action. He postulated that a therapeutic community under-
goes oscillations of social integration and that there were
times when the administration could be passive and let the
patients run things and other times when the explosive forces
threatened disintegration. When this happened the doctors
had to act. In any therapeutic community the leaders – the
staff group and in particular the doctor and the head nurse –
will have to be flexible; they will hand over as much power as
possible, but will take firm action if there is a crisis, and then
hand over again when it has passed.

In all human administrative roles the judgement of timing
and intensity of internal regulative action is a major function
of leadership – when to punish transgressors and when to
ignore them, when to be firm, when to be weak, when to
'assert authority'. The fact that nearly every novel of cor-
porate life involves this theme shows that it is an area of
difficulty for all. But psychiatrists have more difficulties than
most here. Doctors in general are action-oriented; they are

trained to 'do something' in times of crisis; psychotherapists are passivity-oriented; they expect to refrain from action and make interpretative comments only. Every psychiatrist is torn between these two roles and many are inhibited or guilty about taking firm action.

A visitor to a noted therapeutic community witnessed an example of permissiveness that had become abdication of responsibility. At the community meeting the women started complaining of a Mr T, who, they said, persisted in using their toilets. It was clear that this was no new topic, but that feeling was rising higher. As they were speaking of him Mr T minced in, dressed in a frock, high heels, and nylons. The patients asked him why he had dressed thus; he said he preferred it. They asked the doctor to do something about the matter; the doctor commented that everyone seemed very angry and he wondered why. The women answered that they did not like men using their lavatories and called for medical action. The doctor again commented on the strength of their feeling. The women questioned Mr T, who said he would stop it if the doctor told him to. Finally, after a silence, the doctor told Mr T that he should dress in his proper clothes. Mr T left the room amidst an outburst of applause and rejoined the meeting ten minutes later dressed in shirt and jeans.

At the subsequent staff meeting the visitor asked about the matter, and precipitated a vigorous discussion. Everyone had been very worried about T and his behaviour; the nurses knew how upset the women patients were but said nothing because, they said, they believed that the doctors approved of this. The doctor said that he did not think it was any help to T to be allowed thus to act out his transvestite fantasies but that he had been waiting for the staff or the patients to speak. He did not wish to be authoritarian.

The visitor felt that the whole episode showed abdication of responsibility; doctors, nurses, and patients had slithered into the situation while waiting for someone else to act. Had it been part of a plan to help T it would have been comprehensible, but no one contended that it would be helpful to him. One effect was to feed the rumours which already circulated about the unit and to increase the hostility to its work.

Sanctions and Rewards

In the old mental hospital wards, punishment was openly discussed. There was a range of penalties for misbehaviour starting from withdrawal of privileges and passing through seclusion, restraint, wet packs, to ECT and leucotomy. When staff became more sophisticated they became ashamed of the ward 'punishment' and would explain that the procedure was therapeutic, that it was being done for the patients' own good. Few of the patients appeared to believe this. In the open community it should be possible to discuss some of the process of control and 'bad' behaviour openly.

Sanctions and rewards are part of the fabric of social life. As soon as people live together there has to be control of behaviour; desired behaviour is rewarded, undesirable behaviour is discouraged. One of the most useful methods of social learning is to see reward or discouragement meted out to other people who are doing what you yourself had a mind to do. We need therefore have no qualms or guilt about saying that our therapeutic community is going to teach its members certain kinds of behaviour, and that we shall encourage and reward desired behaviour and discourage undesirable behaviour. The first reason is that the community may continue to exist and not disintegrate. But that was why the attendants used to beat up the violent patients – so that they would not kill them or the other patients. Their method was fairly successful in turning homicidal madmen into docile asylum chronics, using the resources of a very small, underpaid, untrained staff. The disadvantage of the method, aside from its inhumanity and brutality, was that it produced a state of social crippling, of institutionalization, which filled the asylums. Our aim is to prepare the patients for discharge. This means a much more complex and flexible system of sanctions and rewards, by which behaviour which threatens community disintegration – such as frequent attacks on other patients – is checked, while lively initiative – even if directed against the established authority – is rewarded and encouraged.

Much of this can be worked out in the community meetings and much internal discipline can be taken over by them. The patients will at first tend to be too punitive of people who offend but will gradually learn to search for the causes of the behaviour. Most of the time the task of the community leaders will be to lead the community to examine aberrant behaviour – why it disturbs them, whether it really harms anybody, what are the reasons for the person committing it.

But these things are difficult to talk about, and this, being an area of uneasiness, is one in which collusion easily develops. If the nurses see that the doctor does not like being asked why he uses ECT, they will stop asking; if the patients are criticized for raising certain problems, they may stop doing so. It is part of the leadership task to be particularly ready to discuss sanctions and rewards and why activities are discouraged. This is a touchy area where the doctor's guilts and anxieties are central because he is the only member of the staff team entrusted by society with the ultimate sanctions. In a neurosis unit it is the doctor who orders patients' discharge, removal by the police, committal to a mental hospital. In a mental hospital it is the doctor alone who can order massive tranquillization, seclusion, electroplexy, leucotomy. Every sensitive doctor will feel guilty about ordering these procedures to control a patient whose behaviour offends him, but he will find that the rest of the staff share many of these guilts and anxieties.

Since, in the wider sense, our society is in constant doubt about how to control deviant behaviour – witness the constant arguments about corporal and capital punishment, prisons, law courts, etc. – it is hardly surprising that this theme constantly recurs in the hospital. The important thing is to discuss it openly and honestly, again and again, and relate action to the need to help the patient toward rehabilitation and discharge and to protect the community from disintegration.

The rewards, too, must be considered. What behaviour is applauded? There is a tendency for nursing staff to prefer passive conforming behaviour and to discourage initiative – yet this may be more helpful towards the individual's rehabilitation. It is always valuable, though sometimes appallingly revealing, to steer conversation towards what the patients feel are the grounds for the allotment of privileges or social rewards such as weekend trips, day passes, ward moves.

Barrier Adjustments
The traditional mental hospital had a tremendously effective barrier – physical, social, psychological – cutting it off from the outer world. Goffman in particular has explored the hospital's stripping procedures, its bizarre rituals, and the

71

great difficulty for anyone – patients or staff – to pass in and out. Such a barrier is almost entirely detrimental, and to a great extent it can be modified by the complaints that come up in the community meetings and the proposals that are made. All the curious admission procedures will be questioned and can be reconsidered. All unnecessary deviations from life outside should be removed and all unnecessary difficulties about going in and out. But the therapeutic community is not life outside. It is a place to which people come when they cannot manage life outside. For some it may be indeed an asylum. For some, a period of respite from their relatives may be as necessary as it is for others to have the reassurance of daily contact with outside reality. Each difference can be examined for its effect on the community life and on certain individual patients.

MAINTENANCE OF THE THERAPEUTIC COMMUNITY

Once the channels of communication have been opened, group discussion and decision-making accepted, the authority pyramid flattened, mutual examination of roles and functions initiated, and the free examination of all happenings well accepted, much has been achieved. But the work goes on.

New problems constantly emerge. Sivadon[50] once remarked that it was good that there was always something wrong in a hospital, since this could be used as the starting-point for joint problem-solving. Even if the community began to reach an efficient and effective state, the new entrants – the new patients with their distressing problems, the new staff with their adjustment difficulties – would provide a constant flow of problems. Mostly there is no need to seek subjects for discussion and consideration; they present themselves. There are, however, subjects to which the administrative therapist can profitably turn his mind occasionally.

Communications

Communications systems are like the bed of the Mississippi as Mark Twain described it – the channels silt up until a flood comes and cuts new channels, which silt up in their course. Any group that comes together has a period of excited sharing of information, experience, and attitudes and then the exchange may become ritualized. This may be the time to dissolve the group, or change its function. It is well to ask any meeting occasionally why it continues to meet. When a new problem arises it is often better to assemble a new *ad hoc* grouping to deal with it rather than to use a pre-existing body; the new group can disperse when the job is done. One sign of silting communications is when someone fails to hear about something of direct importance to him. This should be taken seriously and the administrative therapist will learn to inquire vigorously at these times. Often major collusions, communication blockages, and misunderstandings will be revealed.

Scanning

The administrative therapist has the general task of scanning the operations of the unit. In any society there will always be neglected corners where things are going wrong. At the ward level, for example, people may be cutting the P.T. classes, curious night-time sessions may be starting, relatives may be turned away by the hospital porter, telephone calls lost. At the hospital level, the kitchens may get dirty, a ward become demoralized, the black market in sedatives extend widely, or strange parties be held in the staff quarters. These are signs of disorganization which, if ignored, may lead to major trouble and disaster. Most of these things will emerge of themselves in a free communication system, but the administrative therapist should also be scanning for them, as others may lack the experience to see things beginning to go wrong, or to spot the first signs of malfunction. Parkinson,[41] has described as 'ingelititis' the state of sagging morale and inefficiency in an organization; the wise administrative therapist will pick up, often subconsciously, the first signs of injelititis, as the experienced clinician will detect a faltering in the pulse. There are different styles of reacting to something being amiss. If the administrative therapist immediately takes action, draws attention to the fault, and asks for explanations, he is working back to the old fault-finding authority that so paralysed the traditional hospital, and is making himself into a feared authority. If there is a fuss when the doctor sees something amiss, one solution is to hide things when the doctor comes by. It may be better to take note but keep silent. Then, when a remark in a meeting offers an opening, the doctor can steer the discussion in that direction. If it emerges that no one else feels anything amiss, he should reconsider his observation; but often he will uncover the problem and the group will then be able to work toward improvement.

Long-Term Planning and Research

Every society has at times to consider its long-term future. For many members of the community this is not a matter of personal interest: the patients hope to be away soon; many staff have only temporary commitments. A review of many wards or hospitals will show that very few of the present members were there three years before, or expect to be there three years from now. There falls, therefore, on the few senior members who admit their permanent commitment the need to think of the future. They should be keeping diaries, maintaining records of admissions and discharges, organizing follow-up studies, planning research programmes. If there are any questions of new buildings, they may have to give many hours to architects and planners.

CHAPTER 5

Positions for Administrative Therapy

Every psychiatrist treating inpatients in an institution ought to be giving some of his time and thought to the administrative therapy of his patients – to the organizing of their lives towards recovery – but what he can do depends on the position he holds; each position in the social system offers some opportunities but imposes certain limitations. By studying the three positions of junior doctor in charge of a ward, senior psychiatrist in charge of a team or division, and medical superintendent, we can see most of the possibilities for administrative therapy. This chapter discusses the situation of a doctor in each of these positions who is attempting to make the social system of the unit help actively towards the patients' recovery.

THE WARD DOCTOR

The doctor who can give most of his time to a single ward is in an excellent position to undertake administrative therapy. The unit is small and clearly defined; staff and patients know one another; he has medical charge of the patients and can control drugs and treatment. Unfortunately, the doctors in this position are often just starting in psychiatry. This is in some ways an advantage as they are not yet inured to hospital ways and their vigour is fed by indignation and pity;

but they lack experience and do not know where to begin. Often, too, they lack knowledge of psychiatry or skill in psychotherapy and may find such tasks as conducting ward meetings very difficult.

The ward doctor will assess the limitations set on his unit by society as a whole but, more important, by the hospital of which it is part. What do they expect from him? What is the unit's task within the hospital? How much will they be allowed to experiment? Most important to him are the attitudes of his medical superiors, in particular the medical superintendent. Many will permit experiment but the test tends to come when the social changes produce repercussions. For the ward doctor the best superintendent is one who lets him make his changes, who tells him of external repercussions but lets the ward work out its answers and who backs them up against unwarranted attack.

Within the British National Health Service, since 1960, clinical responsibility rests with the consultant psychiatrist. If he acts as ward doctor, the situation is clear. If all the patients are under the responsibility of one consultant and he gives the ward doctor full support, then the situation is reasonable. But the fairly common situation where several different consultants with different notions of treatment have patients in one ward, makes the development of a therapeutic community very difficult. Even when they give formal consent to social restructuring, they will be surprised and probably indignant when they find doctors, nurses, and patients departing from their traditionally prescribed behaviour, and, for instance, other patients suggesting changes in drug dosage. Many young administrative therapists in Britain have found this their greatest sphere of difficulty, though a number have overcome the problems and set up effective therapeutic communities.

A registrar at a mental hospital became interested in social psychiatry and read several books on therapeutic communities. He had completed his training appointments in the hospital and had passed his D.P.M. (Board) examinations. His next assignment was to a 'convalescent' ward for women; he approached the medical superintendent who had expressed general interest in these ideas and asked permission to run the ward as a therapeutic community. He had talks with the matron, the ward sister, the nursing tutor, and each of the senior psychiatrists about what he hoped to do.

He reorganized the ward around community meetings, small group meetings, and frequent staff discussions. The experiment went well. The patients stopped grumbling about the food and began to talk about their feelings about one another and the staff, their fears and anxieties, and began openly to face their desire for dependence and fears of discharge. The staff began to discuss their own dissensions and disagreements, to criticize one another, and to modify some of their professional rigidities. The ward became a much livelier, though untidier place; the staff and patients on the ward, with some hesitations, welcomed the changes.

The repercussions from the rest of the hospital were sharp. His fellows among the junior doctors criticized the disorder and the fact they were called down at nights about rows between the patients. They also pointed out to him that he was wasting his time with this stuff when he might be pursuing his career. Other senior nurses were very critical of the ward sister. Rumours ran round the hospital that the place encouraged unethical practices among the nurses. Patients on other wards were unwilling to be transferred to the unit. Some senior psychiatrists said that their special patients were being unduly disturbed. The medical superintendent veered uneasily between asking to attend ward meetings and ostentatiously washing his hands of the 'goings on' at staff conferences. Just before the Hospital Open Day the matron came on the ward in the doctor's absence, criticized the untidiness (the result of an agreed staff policy of letting the patients work through a problem of cleansing rotas), and instructed the ward sister and the nurses to clean the place up. When a fire in the ward (possibly deliberate) was so severe that the fire brigade had to be called and the Hospital Management Committee informed, the anxieties welled highest and there was nearly a formal inquiry.

Ultimately the experiment was successful. Two years later all applauded it. The patients preferred the new way of things and made better recoveries; the nurses became enthusiastic and other wards copied the pattern. The registrar's own position prospered; papers were presented to conferences and published. Looking back, however, the doctor recalled the early months as some of the loneliest he had ever had. Surprised by the depth and intensity of the patients' anxieties, criticized by his fellows, under pressure, overt and covert from his seniors, the nurses alternately criticizing him and begging for reassurance, he often doubted his inspiration.

In retrospect it seemed that certain factors had been important in sustaining him and the ward against the criticism and hostility and saving the experiment from collapse. He was well known, well liked, and well respected through the hospital; the senior psychiatrists trusted him to handle their patients with sense and discretion, the nurses and the other ward doctors were at least prepared to suspend judgement for a time. The medical superintendent's ambivalences also helped; his desire to be thought 'permissive' balanced his anxieties about what was going on in a part of 'his' hospital; his general commitment to social psychiatry inhibited his impulse to interfere in the name of administrative efficiency.

The assessment of a ward's potentialities is comparatively easy. The type of patient is usually fairly well defined, as well as the function of the ward. A ward has usually a given task within the total organization of the hospital and this will indicate possible lines of development. For a 'convalescent' ward the aim could be more rapid and effective discharges; for an admission ward, less stressful initiation and more rapid return home; for a 'wet and dirty' ward, the elimination of incontinence; for a 'refractory' ward, the elimination of restraint, the development of self-government and internal regulation, and possibly opening the ward door.

The staff group is small; the key people are the charge nurse or charge attendant and the deputies. The doctor can first win their confidence and trust by attending to the requests and problems they bring forward and then discuss with them how the ward could perhaps do its job better. Their goodwill is essential. They have seen doctors come and go. If a doctor shows more interest than usual in the life of the ward, they will fear that he is a troublemaker, out to get them fired, or worse, that he is going to rouse their hopes with new plans and then move away, leaving them to clean up as others have done before. Their first reaction will therefore be hesitant and guarded. The doctor will be able to initiate little until he has won their confidence to some extent, at least. This he can first do by ordinary medical competence, by doing promptly and effectively the medical tasks they bring to him.

The rest of the ward staff and the other professional staff should all be seen and assessed. Are they competent? Are there any untapped sources of energy? Often there will be one or two among them who will be obvious sources of energy – a nursing assistant who has 'always wanted to do more'; a social worker who has read about therapeutic communities; an aide who is attending college and wonders if he could ever become a nurse. The patients' group may contain some effective personalities; particularly in a long-stay ward in a hospital where there have not been many discharges, certain patients may be key members of the ward life and important culture-carriers. Once he has won the respect of the senior nurses, the doctor should try to see something of the ward life by visiting at different times and staying about the ward; this will worry them but if done with care can be acceptable. Invitations to take tea or coffee on the ward, to attend a party, to inspect some faulty plumbing or damaged furniture are often good points of entry and provide ways of demonstrating an interest in the ward life beyond the strict medical role.

From these sources a picture of the social life of the ward will emerge with possible points for improvement and goals that might be achieved.

Timing is important in the next stages. The staff and patients will realize that this is a different sort of doctor; they will be excited and hopeful, anxious and alarmed. His aim is to maintain hope yet allay suspicion while he brings first the staff, then the whole ward, together. If he plunges in and calls a ward meeting without consultation, it will probably fail disastrously. The staff will sit in glowering silence while he attempts vainly to deal with the storms that arise; then somehow the arrangements for the next meeting will fall through – the nurses will be off duty, or all the patients will be on bath parade, or ward stocks have to be checked; before long the meeting will be just a bad memory. The best starting-point is a common problem or project. Something will crop up – a difficult patient to deal with, a ward outing to plan, a rearrangement of timetables and he can get the staff together to discuss it. If it goes well he can suggest further meetings and then regular ones. In these, sooner or later, junior staff will challenge their seniors; here he must give support both in the meeting and afterwards, so as to keep everyone in the team. It is in these meetings that occupational therapists and social workers, volunteers, ward orderlies, and others can be brought into the team. The doctor is chairman of this meeting and he must learn to act effectively and wisely. He should refrain from too much lecturing and try to bring in the con-tributions of all, especially the junior, shy, or tongue-tied members. If a problem occurs that warrants it, the head nurse, the director of nursing education, or the clinical director can be asked to attend. This gives status to the meet-ing and gives these administrators an idea of the ward's problems.

Once the staff meetings are established, an opportunity to call a ward meeting will present iself. This should be fully prepared, as the nurses and attendants may feel threatened. They may have heard tales of ward meetings: how the patients criticize the nurses while the doctor sits smiling; how all ward discipline is destroyed. The whole social struc-ture and their system of control is being challenged, and though they may welcome the possibility of change, they will still be frightened. A staff meeting should be held immediately after the ward meeting in order to work through these legi-timate anxieties.

By all these moves, the communication structure is radi-cally altered. The doctor hears direct from the patient or the attendant about what happened, rather than at second or third hand. As the staff group start to work together authority patterns change; they may decide on a plan of action for a patient and delegate one attendant to carry it out; as the junior nurses hear the doctor explain the treatment policy they become bolder in doing what they think will be helpful. The occupational therapist finds herself much more accepted and can link her activities with those of the nursing staff; the social worker brings a clear picture of the families and their problems to the staff and also has a better picture of the patients' behaviour to inform her talks with the relatives.

Over a period of months the new pattern will be established. The meetings will be accepted and used by patients and staff to solve the ward's problems; they will have their ups and downs – some dreary and dull, others lively and productive. Staff members will come to understand one another's work better and begin to appreciate others' personalities, abilities, and failings.

Sooner or later, something will go wrong; something involving the outside – the rest of the hospital. This will be the testing time. A patient will run away, get drunk, start a fight, commit suicide; the director of nursing will see an attendant sitting chatting with the patients and tell the charge nurse that he should be polishing the door knobs; the hospital engineer will complain to the medical superintendent that too many windows are being broken; a long-term nurse will resign and give the 'disorganization' of the ward as her reason; the nursing tutor will complain that attendants are being allowed to do nurses' jobs, or nurses asked to do attendants' jobs. The common factor in these examples is that an important and powerful figure in the hospital has received a complaint arising from the new way of running the ward. This will be a chance for hostile and critical people to bring pressure to bear on the ward and the doctor to 'stop all this nonsense'.

Much will depend on how the doctor acts. He is the spokesman of the ward team; all the ward, and much of the hospital, will be watching. He will have to defend, explain, protest, and cajole. It may be easiest to see this as a battle against forces of reaction, in which he is a knight fighting dragons; so long as it helps him to battle, such simple notions are good. It is not, however, so important that he wins the battle, as how he fights; even a defeat can be helpful to the ward, if it is a spur to them to win the next time. What matters is the result within the ward, in the feelings of the staff and the patients. The doctor's prime objectives should be to strengthen, unite, and reassure his ward therapeutic team, to demonstrate his commitment and loyalty to them and the joint project, and if possible to convince the rest of the hospital that what they are doing is worth while. The patients and staff of the ward must feel that the doctor is not going to abandon them.

Of the leadership tasks the ward doctor will probably find the group-conducting the most challenging. For many patients, especially English patients, it is a new experience to be a member of an unstructured meeting of thirty or forty people; certainly very few will have ideas of how to proceed and act. The meeting will have to evolve its own traditions of how much activity or comment is permissible, how vigorous personal interpretations should be, how much it looks to the doctor to say all the wise things, or the head nurse to state all the regulations.

Goal-setting comes naturally in staff discussions; sanctions and rewards are easily discussed in a ward meeting; barrier adjustments will be a major matter of discussion for many months.

There will be a great deal of role discussion and definition once the therapeutic community is well established. Many functions will change and there will be long talks and many feelings about this, The patients will take over much of the work; they will assume responsibility for much maintenance work and also for some internal regulation, possibly reprimand of offenders and fitness for leave. The attendants and assistant nurses, freed of housework, will be talking and interacting with patients – more interesting but more taxing work. The charge nurse will find his position changing; he will be more of a teacher and adviser and less of an executive.

The doctor's work will also have become much richer and more fascinating. The patients will no longer be just cases – 'chronic dements' – 'typical epileptics' – but people with hopes and fears, whom he has seen through storms and achievements. He will find that being a member of a therapeutic community is perplexing and at times disturbing, as when his pronouncements are queried or discarded in public by patients or staff, or when his motives are publicly challenged, but that it is far more interesting and that he is far closer to the feelings and needs of the patients than ever before.

The examination of roles is an essential part of the development of a therapeutic community; everyone is interested in the work of others and for a number of months explores them. Then comes a period of clarification and definition. After seeing how much everyone has in common, the group begins to examine what each has that is different. The work of the doctor, among others, is examined. They have seen that he too can become a member of the therapeutic community, that he can contribute to understanding people, that he reacts warmly to others' problems, that he too is

85

fallible and emotional; that he is not a god-like individual with much secret knowledge. Now they begin to assess what are the special contributions that he makes because of his long, specialized, expensive, professional education.

His skilled contributions can be grouped thus. He is a medical doctor, a psychiatrist, a member of the hospital medical staff, an expert on psychodynamics and on social psychiatry, and an educated citizen. In the average psychiatric ward there is not a great deal of physical medicine called for and most of it is minor; any major illness is usually treated in a special department. His medical knowledge will, however, often be called on, sometimes legitimately and sometimes defensively, in ward discussions. His psychiatric knowledge of diagnosis and prognosis can be very important in an admitting unit; in a long-stay unit is is less important, and senior nurses and psychologists may know as much or more than he. This is often a source of anxiety to the doctor who is fairly new to psychiatry.

The doctor has certain powers, granted by law or by the hospital, which are of value to the ward community. Only he can order potent drugs, sign death certificates, order ECT, or detain a patient; he is usually the only staff member who can arrange admissions and discharges. At times this may cause him difficulties when the team press him to perform some act, such as ordering ECT, for which he will be personally, legally responsible. He may have to discuss these responsibilities quite openly with them. As a doctor he is a member of the most powerful status group in the hospital; his concurrence in decisions lends great strength to them and is useful to the team.

The therapeutic community needs someone to help it to understand the significance of emotional happenings. Though intuition and native wit can see a lot, all therapeutic com-

munities to date have included several people with analytic
or psychotherapeutic knowledge or experience. The group
tends to look to the doctor for this, and it may be difficult for
a relatively junior doctor to meet that need. Sometimes a
clinical psychologist can meet it better.

The group also need someone with knowledge of social
psychiatry – of what other therapeutic communities have
done, and how they have got on. They need someone who
has read the books and the discussions, and if possible someone who has visited or worked in other therapeutic communities. This again may come in part from other staff members,
but is often supplied by the doctor.

Finally, the doctor has usually had the most expensive
education of any of the ward community; he is one of the few
college graduates in it. As a result he will be called on for information and opinions on many subjects of law and life,
though he should beware of becoming too much of an
'expert'.

One of the problems that faces the administrative therapist
on the ward is that the staff will tend to take him for a model
in some of their actions. This may be appropriate in, for
instance, the analysis of motivation and the unravelling of the
causes of some happenings in the ward. But there are other
spheres where he is lacking in knowledge and should not
allow himself to be used as a model, such as the proper way
to handle patients when they are deeply disturbed or violent.
This is something for which his medical training has not
prepared him and he is far less well equipped to deal with
this than experienced nurses. This is an occasion for humility, when he can learn, can watch how they approach the
problem, and realize how much other skills than his own are
needed for the team.

Another sphere of medical ignorance is how the patients

live at home. Many hospital doctors make recommendations that reveal their ignorance of working-class living conditions. The social worker, the attendants, and the other patients can often advise far better than the doctors in this area.

The classic description of administrative therapy from the position of ward doctor is Wilmer's[56] account of the Naval admitting ward. He did this work from the position of ward doctor, but with a considerable background of experience. In 1955, when he went to Oakland, he had been medically qualified for fifteen years, had been trained in psychiatry and in psycho-analysis and had had experience of therapeutic community work with Maxwell Jones.

THE SENIOR PSYCHIATRIST

The position of senior psychiatrist in charge of a division of a mental hospital or a psychiatric unit in a general hospital frequently offers opportunities for administrative therapy. Although not a very satisfying position within mental hospitals in the past, the development of the concepts of clinical teams and of decentralization has improved the position of the senior psychiatrist and it has been further strengthened in England by the Mental Health Act 1959. This gave the 'responsible medical officers' (senior psychiatrists usually of 'consultant' grade) complete legal and clinical responsibility for their patients. If he has the inclination, the senior psychiatrist is now in a very favourable position to do administrative therapy. He has the psychiatric experience, the status within the hospital, the legal responsibility, and long-term commitment which the ward doctor often lacks, while he is free of many of the diverse commitments of the medical superintendent.

The senior psychiatrist will have stable relations with the

senior nursing, medical, and lay staff in the hospital and should be respected by them. This will make it much easier to maintain the therapeutic community against interference and to defend it against criticism. He has less need to persuade, since he has the ultimate legal responsibility for the treatment of his patients and thus the right to attempt to replan their way of life.

His assessment is also easier; his main problem will be to decide whether to concentrate on one ward or to spread his effort over several. If he concentrates on one ward his problems and procedures will be those discussed in the last section. To apply administrative therapy to a whole division will benefit more patients, but will be more complex. The boundaries of his authority are important, for it is in areas of disputable authority that difficulties may arise. If he shares facilities on a ward, such as an admission unit, with several other senior psychiatrists who prefer the traditional routine, then it will be difficult to do much to change the lives of his patients there. It is very difficult to organize a therapeutic milieu for one-third of the patients on a ward and not for the others. If patients of other psychiatrists are on his wards, he should come to an understanding with them; otherwise they may instruct the nurses to adopt attitudes or give treatment in a manner that conflicts with what is done for the other patients and he may find himself being challenged in the open ward meeting about medical instructions with which he does not agree but which he feels he should defend. The area of nursing authority is vital, and he must come to an understanding with the head nurse before he starts. If he is going to reorganize the life of a division of the hospital – and inevitably the work of the nurses – he needs a senior nursing officer whose main work will be with him and his unit, and who is responsible for the nursing practices in the unit. Any other arrangement leads to great difficulties, because the main hospital nursing administration has so many other (legitimate) interests to take heed of.

The course of action is again essentially the same. Opening up communications is the first step; he can call together staff groups to consider unit problems. From these will emerge difficulties and tasks to tackle and he can gradually bring in the other necessary people – social workers, occupational therapists, psychologists. From these meetings, the idea of patients' meetings will in due course develop.

The senior psychiatrist inevitably works more with staff and less directly with patients than the ward doctor. He will probably have some doctors working under him and his relationship with them is, of course, very important. They will be under his authority and it may be his task to train them in psychiatry.

You cannot direct a person to do administrative therapy any more than you can order a convinced organic therapy enthusiast to carry out psychotherapy; there must be a desire and a capacity to learn. Some may be unwilling to do some of the simpler tasks of administrative therapy such as con-ducting a patients' meeting and others may be incapable of doing them. If there is a rotation system of training, there may not be time for doctors to learn the ways of the thera-peutic community or become useful before they are moved on. After assessment, the senior psychiatrist may decide that for some doctors it is better to remain in the uncommitted traditional medical role than to risk the pains of involvement. As the work spreads, he will find junior doctors asking to come on the unit and willing to spend time learning the techniques. These are the ones with whom he can really work and one of his tasks will be training them. He can encourage them to sit in on the community meetings, to deputize for him when he is away, and then to discuss how they handled the problems that arose.

Of the leadership tasks mentioned, he will have to undertake many. He will be particularly concerned with 'barrier mechanics', as he will control – or be able to influence – admission and discharge policies of the unit. He will also be able to undertake activities with mental health associations and volunteers' organizations to bring in outside help and to make the rehabilitation process less difficult. He can give his mind to long-term planning and research. There is not enough examination and analysis of the procedures, successes, and failures of administrative therapy. A senior psychiatrist can make approaches to research foundations for funds to support social scientists who are studying programmes. He can arrange for the collection of data and records, the analysis of trends, and the recording of meetings.

The spokesman function will of course be important when the inevitable outside difficulties and repercussions flow back on to the unit, and goal-setting and slogan-choosing will be among his major functions.

Some of the studies of therapeutic communities were written by administrative therapists who worked from the position of senior psychiatrist.

Martin was a consultant psychiatrist at Claybury during the period described in his book, although he became medical superintendent shortly afterwards.

Maxwell Jones's position at Belmont was that of a consultant psychiatrist responsible for a separate unit. Some of Rapoport's[49] discussions illustrate administrative therapy principles, and the doctor's role: 'Oscillations in the State of Social Organization' (p. 135) illustrates the principle of flexibility of authority; 'The Role of Junior Psychiatrist' (p. 111) illustrates some of the problems of the entering doctor. Unfortunately, Maxwell Jones's own pivotal and creative role in the unit is not examined.

THE MEDICAL SUPERINTENDENT

When psychiatric institutions began a century and a half ago, the medical superintendents were the administrative therapists, undertaking responsibility for every part of the administration of the asylum in order to develop a healthy atmosphere for the patients. They called this 'moral treatment' and contrasted it with the usual medical activity of giving pills and potions. Physicians were appointed as medical superintendents and given supreme authority over all other officers in the asylum in order to ensure that the needs of the patients were kept paramount. Regrettably, over the century the vision was lost; there are a number of reasons, but one was the failure of the doctors themselves to remember this part of their work as they became involved in morbid pathology or 'disease' classification or hygiene and sanitation; their enthusiasm for moral treatment wilted as they became convinced of the hereditary degeneracy of insanity, the inevitability of the dementia of dementia praecox, or the overriding necessity for secure custody for long-term patients.

The medical superintendent of the moral treatment hospitals of the early nineteenth century was the only medical officer to about two hundred patients; he was ward doctor, senior psychiatrist, and medical superintendent combined; he had legal responsibility for all of them and power to rearrange the life of the hospital to fit their needs. It was an ideal situation for administrative therapy and this is probably why good results were frequently achieved. Nowadays only a few doctors are in this position – the directors of private sanatoria, or the medical superintendents of very small public mental hospitals. It is interesting that the first open-door hospital had this pattern. Dingleton Hospital had only 400 patients and Dr Bell knew them all personally when he opened the doors in 1949.

Unfortunately in most mental hospitals it became more and more difficult for the medical superintendent to practise administrative therapy even if he had the inclination. The hospitals were made bigger and bigger, until they contained thousands of patients, from whom the medical superintendent was very remote. He still was legally responsible for all of them and for all the running of the hospital. Individual treatment was necessarily in the hands of other members of the medical staff; the medical superintendent often had no patients of his own, sometimes (in the United States) was not a psychiatrist, and frequently functioned more as a medically qualified business administrator and committee man. Any good milieu therapy was a triumph against almost overwhelming difficulties of size and legal restrictions.

During the last twenty years the position of the medical superintendent has developed differently in England and in the United States. In the United States he is still personally responsible for the custody and treatment of all the patients and is fully responsible for all the details of the running of the hospital; it is very difficult for him to undertake administrative therapy. In England, mental hospitals never became so huge. The medical superintendent was relieved of responsibility for the business administration in 1948 and of the legal responsibility for all the patients in 1959. The medical superintendent is now one of a group of senior psychiatrists who are fairly equal in status and pay. He is clinically and legally responsible only for those patients under his personal care. There is, in fact, no legal necessity for an English mental hospital in the 1960s to have a medical

93

superintendent, and some have instead a Medical Staff Committee with a chairman whose term of office is limited. In most mental hospitals, however, the post of medical superintendent has been retained and the psychiatrist who holds it is entrusted by his consultant colleagues with the general task of co-ordinating the therapeutic activities of the hospital. The Ministry of Health recognized this by defining the medical superintendent as 'the chief officer of the hospital for the therapeutic sphere'. Administrative therapy is the task of such men and a tremendous opportunity.

The medical superintendent's position gives a senior psychiatrist far more power to change the hospital. He is in direct and daily contact with the officers who control the material side of the hospital's life and employ many of the patients – the secretary, the engineer, the catering officer, the farm manager; he works regularly and closely with the chief nursing officers; he has direct access to the granters of funds and facilities – Management Committees or State Commissioners of Hygiene. He has also direct contact with the public volunteer groups, Rotary Clubs, Townswomen's Guilds, Soroptimists, etc., and organs of public opinion – press, radio, etc. – who become accustomed to taking note of what he says. It is comparatively easy, therefore, for the medical superintendent to bring about dramatic changes in the life of the hospital. His very power, however, is a disadvantage. It makes the staff defer to him, especially as he gets older and possibly wiser; it is easy for staff, doctors and nurses, to slip into a subservient, dependent-hostile relationship to him which not only stunts them but contributes to re-establishing that traditional asylum atmosphere which so crippled the patients' independence and initiative. One of the great dangers to a medical superintendent and the hospital he serves arises if he has too lively a mind, if he has too many

94

bright ideas, especially if they are mostly good ones. They are accepted; and gradually the staff stop thinking for themselves; they just wait for the next instructions. The good administrative therapist should create an atmosphere where other people have ideas, where other people feel the urge to offer proposals and are given the chance to work them out. The ideas of nurses, junior doctors, and patients may often be more helpful than the superintendent's ideas, because they are in direct contact with the patients on the wards; but that is not so important as the fact that emerging ideas are evidence of an atmosphere that encourages self-expression, initiative, and personal development and it is such an atmosphere that the patient needs so much.

The assessment task is fairly easy for the administrative therapist in the medical superintendent's post. He has access to all the data of staff and patient categories, histories, methods of entry, etc. He knows most of the staff. The only danger is that he knows only those aspects of people which they wish to show him.

Many staff remember the old days when the medical superintendent had great power over nearly everyone and was a person to be feared, shunned, placated, or hated according to one's temperament. Even now his power to discharge nurses, to give doctors bad references, to detain patients, are great enough to make most staff careful what they show him of themselves. Even if he is a mild benign man who never uses these powers, he is the head of the system, and the focus of everyone's unresolved Oedipal fantasies; he will find himself credited with magical prescience or malignant tyranny however ordinary his actions.

In the old days many hospitals had elaborate warning systems of the medical superintendent's movements, telephone calls, pipe-tapping systems, sentinel patients who shouted when he approached, so important was it to ensure that he did not know too much. The superintendent's attempts to assess the hospital or the people in it will therefore always be limited. Sometimes the judgement of a man's peers may be a better measure of his worth than the face he shows to the superintendent.

The action to be taken in changing the milieu is essentially similar, though the superintendent will work almost entirely through staff and seldom directly with patients. Group administrative meetings open communications. Group decisions openly arrived at in the presence of all legitimately interested do much to establish confidence and gain acceptance of common goals. A first point for attention is nearly always the occupation of the patients; what work they do, how much money they get, who pays it out, who gets the work for them. In most hospitals there is scope for the introduction of contract work from factories. Another point for attention is how patients move round the hospital; who moves them from one ward to another, when, and why. This is nearly always an area of conflict, and often of lamentable punitive practices. Meetings of all involved will gradually bring tensions and problems to the surface. Regular meetings are needed of certain key groups in the hospital – the executive officers (secretary, kitchen manager, gardener, head nurses, senior doctors) – the medical staff, senior and junior, the senior nurses, the occupational staff. In all of these he can open communications and develop common goals.

One evening at about 9.0 p.m., a newly appointed medical superintendent met a curious pair walking down a corridor; a junior nurse carrying a bundle of clothing followed by a weeping woman patient, barefoot, in a nightdress. He inquired what was happening and was told the patient had just been awakened from her bed to be moved to another ward, because her bed was needed.

Further inquiries the next morning revealed that an unexpected admission had come late in the evening; since there was no vacant bed in the admission unit, a patient had to be moved to the sick ward; since there was no vacant bed there, a patient had to be transferred to a workers' ward; to make room for her, the patient he had met had had to be awakened from her bed and transferred. Accompanying the unfolding of this tale were many accusations of messages lost or ignored between the doctors and the senior nursing staff.

Appalled by the inhumane results of this sorry tale of overcrowding, misunderstandings, animosities, and blocked communications, he called a meeting of the doctors and administrative nurses involved. He told them what he had seen and suggested that something better should be possible. After the recriminations had subsided it became clear that everyone was in genuine difficulties. Admissions and sudden illnesses were unpredictable and beds very short. The routine for transfers was not clearly defined; patients were moved for medical needs, because of transgression of the rules, or because beds were needed. All concerned were distressed at what they were forced to do, and resentful of the conditions that made it necessary.

Since feelings were so strong he felt this was a good point to start administrative therapy. He proposed daily meetings to consider transfers and ward vacancies; he gave his authority for the setting up enough extra beds to give a margin for manœuvre.

These daily meetings gradually established amicable communications between the medical and administrative nursing staff. Each saw some of the others' problems and anxieties. It was soon ruled that no patient might be transferred without the authority of the joint meeting (except in emergency). Each transfer and the reasons for it were fully discussed. This led to some modification of punitive practices. The nurses gradually drew the doctors' attention to certain patients who seemed fit for discharge.

Over the months the problem became less intense. Transfers were arranged in good time so that there were always vacancies in a crisis. A number of patients were discharged so that the extra beds were taken down. The regular meeting remained as an essential clearing house for medical and nursing problems.

This shows the use of group problem-solving, but there are other notable points. It started from an obviously unsatisfactory situation – so everyone was motivated to examine what they were doing and if necessary to change. It started from the needs of the patients – needs which everyone in the hospital will admit to be overriding.

The authority problem is a major one for the medical superintendent, as we have indicated; his position is in reality fairly powerful, but it is made far more powerful by the fantasies condensed on it. He will want to dispel these and induce a rational approach to himself. Of every task brought to him he can ask, 'Can I not give this to someone else?' 'Could this not be done equally well by someone else?' There is no need for the medical superintendent to decide new colour schemes, to choose new furniture, to plan the layout of new gardens, to be captain of the cricket team, or to be Santa Claus at the Christmas party; all these jobs can be done by other people; they will enjoy doing them, and may do them better than he.

If the job is unpleasant, uncongenial, and difficult, however, he should consider keeping it, for he may be abdicating if he hands it on. But if he holds on to decision-making and insists on referral he does great harm to the atmosphere. An over-anxious medical superintendent, who insists that everything should be referred to him, is one of the most crippling misfortunes that can befall a mental hospital. If the medical superintendent can begin to share responsibility, others will begin to do so too, and ultimately the process will reach the patients – many of whom so badly need more chance to exercise responsibility over part at least of their lives.

Scanning is difficult for the medical superintendent because of the anxiety which traditionally attended superintendents 'tripping' visits to the wards. If he sits in his office all day he will become progressively less well informed about the hospital; but if he inspects and then punishes, people will hide things from him. The best pattern is probably to move around frequently, preferably with some purpose, to notice constantly but to refrain from comment at the time.

Of the leadership tasks, some will seldom fall to him, such as that of interpreter; others can do this better and more fittingly. He will be chairman of many meetings and must learn to be a good chairman-leader, drawing out others' best contributions, but he may not need to conduct therapeutic groups. If he does not already possess experience and ability in the conduct of formal meetings, the rules of procedure, and the proper order of debate, he should take steps to acquire it. There is nothing esoteric about committee procedure – it is just codified common sense to enable people who may be deeply and passionately divided to get through necessary public business without open brawling – but it is well to know the rules of a game before joining it. An

H   99 incompetent chairman is a burden to a meeting; anyone who takes the chair owes it to those who put him there to know the elements of his social task.

His spokesman activities will be many. In Britain, he has to deal with the Hospital Management Committee, a body of local citizens who decide many important questions affecting the hospital's life. They arbitrate among the senior officers, and the medical superintendent must win their approval for any major changes in the life of the hospital. It is before them that he must wage his major battles with the eternal vigilance of the financiers attempting to limit expenditure and to control the workings of the hospital. In the United States, the medical superintendent has to argue with Commissioners of Mental Hygiene and State Treasurers; the forum is different but the arguments are much the same. In both countries he has to be spokesman for the hospital with the public, in the law courts, and at public functions; he has to appear at inquests after suicides; he may have to testify at Inquiries. His remarks will be reported in the papers and will be read not only by the public but also by the staff and patients of the hospital, who will watch to see if he is fighting for the advances that they have made. If he can learn to think on his feet and give clear, prompt, and satisfying answers, he will manage much better; it is fortunately a knack that comes to most with time and practice.

Barrier adjustments are an area where a medical superintendent can do much. If he is frightened and keeps the press out, or is anxious in his public appearances, he increases the stigma on his patients. If he invites the press into the hospital, holds Open Days, fêtes, and gymkhanas he will do much to remove fears. He can talk to groups and encourage volunteer visits; he can speak often to explain modern forms of treatment. He can also take a major part in staff recruitment, which is one of the important means by which new members enter the community.

He can affect greatly sanctions and rewards within the hospital. They are the main social regulating mechanism of the permanent staff and should be part of the mechanism for producing and maintaining a therapeutic atmosphere. For what reasons are staff punished, or rewarded? For what reasons are they promoted or discharged? What reasons do those who make the promotions give for their choices, and, more important, what is believed in the hospital? In every mental hospital there is strong feeling about this; in many there is cynicism and bitterness. The old seniority rule was easy to administer but it put a premium on safe conformity; if you did nothing you would win promotion in the end. A system of promotion by merit is much better, but how and by whom is merit to be assessed? Many devices have been tried, including peer group assessment. The administrative therapist should do all he can to see that promotion goes to those who exert themselves to help patients toward recovery and that only offences against the welfare of the patients or the good of the hospital incur punishment.

One of the medical superintendent's functions is to act as an umbrella over developing projects in the hospital. Junior doctors, ward charge nurses, occupational therapists, and others will want to start projects – redecorating, cooking, outings, special therapeutic groups. The medical superintendent may well foresee, from his experience, difficulties with lay administration, the finance department, and others. He should try not to stop the project because of all the difficulties he can foresee, but guide it in ways that will avoid them. More important, he must shelter the developing project from these adverse criticisms until it is securely established. Sooner or later the critics will have their say; it is important to delay this until the therapeutic value of the idea is established.

The medical superintendent can therefore do a great deal to change things. But to do truly valuable administrative therapy is more difficult. He has somehow to encourage spontaneous change and the emergence of new ideas; he must create an atmosphere where people can disagree with him and push through ideas without his approval, a most difficult task.

One of the penalties of the medical superintendent's position is divorcement from patients. This is hard for the administrative therapist who has gained satisfaction from direct work in therapeutic communities. He will, of course, be meeting patients in hospital, social clubs, and activity groups but it will be difficult for him to be a part of a direct therapeutic team. It may, however, be possible for him to have a ward or a unit of his own where he acts as the senior psychiatrist and thus keeps in touch with a living therapeutic community.

CHAPTER 6

Selection and Training of Administrative Therapists

The analysis of the tasks of the administrative therapist has indicated some of the skills and needs and has suggested some of the qualities desirable. We shall here discuss these further and consider the way by which a person may become a competent administrative therapist. Most good administrative therapists have been medically qualified, trained in psychiatry, experienced in psychotherapy, skilled in group work, and informed about social psychology and social psychiatry. This is a formidable list; fortunately not all are prerequisites, and some can be acquired while practising administrative therapy. We shall consider each.

Medical Training

Most administrative therapists have been doctors. Every therapeutic team must have a medically qualified member. In some Veterans Administration hospitals in the United States good programmes of milieu therapy have been run by clinical psychologists possessing all the other necessary skills, with a doctor providing the drug and treatment facilities as a supporting member of the team. This was also the

Administrative Therapy

position in the early decades of the York Retreat. Jepson ran the house, with William Tuke's support, and the visiting physician was a comparatively minor figure. In general, though, hospitals are reluctant to accept any other than a doctor as the leader of a treatment team.

Psychiatric Training

For senior posts in mental hospitals, formal psychiatric training, the Diploma in Psychological Medicine in England and Board qualification in the United States, is usually required. There have been good administrative therapists without these formal qualifications, but nearly all of them had extensive knowledge and experience of psychiatric illnesses. Certainly a knowledge of psychiatric illnesses, their manifestations, and their outcome, is necessary in dealing with people suffering from them. Some ward doctors attempting administrative therapy have had difficulties because of their lack of psychiatric experience, especially in setting goals too ambitious for crippled people, but there is a greater danger that long experience of the recurring failures of chronic patients may induce too great pessimism.

Psychotherapeutic Experience

This is essential for an understanding of the dynamics of group disturbances, to make useful interpretations, and to have some awareness of one's own reactions. Experience of group psychotherapy is best, as it develops skills of direct value in group meetings and in administration. Most modern administrative therapists have had formal psychotherapeutic training, but it is not certain how necessary a personal analysis is for an administrative therapist; many have had it, many not. By revealing to a man the unconscious roots of his prejudices and showing him his blind spots and weaknesses it will make him less liable to mismanage some of the disturbing material that will emerge in meetings, and may make him more tolerant and accepting of others' sicknesses and weaknesses; his knowledge of his own extra skill may add to his feeling of security.

It is difficult to predict the future here. Most psychiatrists who go through full psycho-analytic training stay in individual therapy – whether because of its fascination, its social worth, or (in the United States) its higher income – and are not available to work with the tens of thousands in institutions who need the help which administrative therapy can give. Yet it is difficult to do administrative therapy without some grounding in psychodynamic theory and some experience in psychotherapy. In some therapeutic communities there may be enough clinical psychologists, social workers, and nurses with psychodynamic training to feed in sufficient awareness without the administrative therapist himself having to supply it. There are increasing opportunities for psychiatrists who do not intend to abandon institutional work to gain psychotherapeutic insight and experience – group therapy, psychotherapy, teaching seminars, a period in personal analysis, individual psychotherapy under supervision – and these may give the extra skill, sensitivity, and insight required. We do not yet know what kind of psychotherapeutic training fits a person best for administrative therapy. Among skilled and justly famous administrative therapists are men who call themselves Adlerians, Jungians, and Sullivanites, men who are fully trained, accredited Freudians, one at least who proclaims himself a failed analysand, and many eclectics.

Group Skills

These can be acquired in the ward and, for many, come easily out of their social experience. Anyone who has been a teacher or an active committee member, a combat officer or a non-commissioned officer, will have acquired enough group skills to start with patient groups. For some doctors, who have not had such experiences, or who are shy or diffident, some preliminary training in small groups may be necessary. An administrative therapist will rapidly acquire these skills, or else give up the work.

Knowledge of Social Psychology and Social Psychiatry
This is mentioned because so few doctors possess it, especially in England. It is as necessary as a knowledge of bio-chemistry is to the practice of medicine. The administrative therapist must prepare himself by a course of reading so that he knows something of the disciplines on which his work is based, and a bibliography is provided on p. 151.

These are the formal qualifications for work as an administrative therapist. What are the desirable personality factors? Can all psychiatrists do this work with equal facility or are some better suited than others? If so, what are the necessary qualities?

This is a difficult problem to discuss. Obviously there are certain qualities desirable in every administrative therapist, just as there are in every doctor, or in every man. Some writers have drawn up lists of estimable qualities in the psychiatric administration; he must have knowledge, skill, intelligence, integrity, maturity, patience, courage, sympathy, farsightedness, etc. Such a list helps us little and merely raises the suspicion that only the Archangel Gabriel (and the compiler of the list) could possibly qualify. On the other hand, administrative therapy is an operation where the therapist's personality and particularly his public manner are his main instruments of therapy; some individuals will be better able to undertake it than others. Taking the list of admirable and desirable human qualities as read, therefore, it seems worth considering those areas of personality functioning which are important in an administrative therapist. These appear to be: attitude to people, feelings about authority and responsibility, social competence, and obsessional anxiety. Every person, by the time he has finished medical training, has fairly settled attitudes in these fields. Some of these promise ease in administrative therapy, others threaten considerable difficulty. We can also indicate areas of competence important in other branches of medicine that do not seem very important in administrative therapy.

Attitude to People
Doctors tend toward two poles of an attitude spectrum – at the one end those who see their patients as individuals and easily become involved in the personal idiosyncrasies of each, and at the other those who regard them as 'cases' and as examples of diseases, and seek to avoid emotional involvement with them. Each pattern of response has been praised and decried. The scientific, logical, detached physician is often esteemed in teaching schools and especially in the preclinical departments, where students are told to value his qualities of clear thinking and his contributions to scientific knowledge. The impersonal approach has advantages, in scientific study, or in surgery of fatal conditions, where too great an emotional involvement could blur judgement. The individual approach, however, is preferred in many practical branches of medicine. Even in medical school the students' own needs take them to the kindly and warm-hearted among their teachers, and patients are notorious for preferring a doctor who responds to them individually and with sympathy. In administrative therapy, as in all psychotherapy,

the personal, emotional attitude toward people is preferable to the impersonal, detached attitude.

Rogers[45] and his group have studied and defined characteristics that make for good psychotherapy. They have shown that, regardless of their formal school of training, therapists with certain characteristics are more effective in helping people. These characteristics are congruent behaviour, a warm, positive acceptant attitude toward the client, and empathic understanding. These attitudes were defined in individual therapy, but they are equally relevant to group or administrative work. Few things annoy a patients' meeting or irritate a committee so much as the sense that the doctor is concealing his feelings, is maintaining a front, is hypocritical, cynical, or 'two-faced', while a willingness on the part of a doctor, or a chairman, to admit and examine his own faults and failings has often been crucial in opening spontaneous developments. Again, in the staff meetings, a feeling that members of one profession can genuinely accept the different standards, attitudes, and values inherent in another is the first step to real trust and teamwork. Experience has shown that those doctors who possess this openness and ability to understand do well in administrative therapy.

Allied with this is the quality seen in the best of teachers – a desire to allow other people to grow – a delight in the development of another. A person who can happily and without envy see a protégé exceed him will do well in administrative therapy. This pleasure in the growth of others is important in individual therapy; it is valuable in the leader of any group, but particularly a group of crippled individuals, battered by many defeats, as the patients in a mental hospital are.

Authority and responsibility

All of us have conflicts and anxieties in this sphere. All of us have unresolved Oedipal difficulties which show themselves at times. Western society, during our lifetime, has seen so many shifts of attitude towards authority that we are all sensitive and easily made anxious on this account. The whole therapeutic community development began with groups of men at odds with all authority (psychopaths) being helped by social psychiatrists sensitive to this area. These conflicts must be moderately resolved before the doctor can function adequately as an administrative therapist. He will do little good if he is absolutely convinced of his suitability to order the lives of others, down to the last detail; but on the other hand he must also be prepared to take responsibility, not be too uncomfortable when authority is laid upon him, and not be so anxious to show his good fellowship that he abdicates from the unpleasant tasks that fall to him. Some of those who enthusiastically embraced the idea of 'therapeutic communities' did so in the hope of getting away from all giving of unpleasant orders. In the therapeutic community, authority may not be such a heavy burden as in the custodial hospital, but responsibility remains.

There are a number of areas of administrative therapy where a person with severe unresolved conflicts about authority and responsibility will get into difficulties. He must be able to delegate, something which is difficult for many doctors, who are accustomed to working on their own and to taking full responsibility only for what they personally do. In administration, delegation is constantly necessary, not only to competent subordinates, but also to incompetent ones. One must learn to leave a subordinate to fumble his way through a job which one could do better oneself; only thus can he learn.

Administrative Therapy

There is a further special area of medical responsibility; we saw that the administrative therapist must be prepared to give medical endorsement to a group decision, for instance to change a patient's medication on the advice of nurses, social workers, or occupational therapists. For some doctors this is most difficult.

Social Competence

To conduct a group calls for a certain readiness of tongue, contact with everything that is happening, and flexibility of response. Most people have enough of this, but some may lack it. The stutterer, the deaf, the very shy will find group work most difficult and might be wise not to attempt it. On the other hand, too complete a social armamentarium can be a disadvantage. The 'commercial traveller', garrulous, overactive, with a quip to meet every contingency, may be so driven by his anxiety to control the social situation that he never has time to listen to what is being said, or to allow the meeting to open up its anxieties. An ability to speak convincingly, allied with the security to keep quiet and listen, is the desirable mean – so seldom achieved.

There is, however, wide scope for individual variation in this area. Each person must work out a style in which he is comfortable and then learn to operate it effectively. Perhaps most important is to establish feedback – to remain sensitive to the reactions to your remarks and behaviour. In all social intercourse we are constantly picking up clues about others' responses to our actions; part of the equipment of a good group leader or committee chairman or lecturer is that he has sharpened this ability in the group situation so that he knows when the group are becoming restless or sleepy, angry or happy, excited or discouraged. He further learns to pick up this information constantly

110

while continuing with his course of action, his talk or his lecture, modifying it as he goes along.

Social skills are fairly easily acquired by most people, and doctors are usually moderately equipped. For the senior roles of administrative therapy they are also valuable; the ability to speak *ex tempore*, to compose 'a few appropriate words' on one's feet, and to give ready answers to unexpected questions are of great value to medical superintendents.

Linked to social competence is political 'toughness' – the ability to get what is necessary, especially from one's superiors. Every administrative therapist has to work within an organization and, as we have noted, has at times to fight for the needs of his patients. Many doctors find the necessary arguing and manoeuvring distasteful (perhaps because they are not good at it) and refuse to involve themselves even in the problems of their own hospital. The man who leads a therapeutic community cannot evade such work. Again, it is a matter of deployment of one's own personality and in particular one's social and verbal aggression. Some work best by making strong demands, striking public attitudes, forcing wordy battles; others achieve more by compromise and the quiet word in the chairman's ear. Most important is the 'reality principle' – the sense of what is practicable, the judgement of what can be achieved. The greatest generals were not those who fought most fiercely but those who did not seek battle unless they had a good chance of victory.

OBSESSIONAL ANXIETY

This is a quality moderately developed in all doctors. In one sphere, that of aseptic theatre routine, it has at one time been intensively developed in all of them. In certain other areas, such as the prescribing of potent drugs or the handling of foodstuffs, they have learned scrupulous exactness. In some parts of administration, notably logistics, the supply department, some obsessional anxiety is valuable; it is good that someone should worry whether everything has been packed. In general medical practice a doctor can hardly be too thorough; but in administrative therapy over-meticulousness can be a grave and even crippling disability. This is particularly clear in the medical superintendent's position; far more hospitals have been damaged by worrying medical superintendents than by slack or dishonest ones. The doctor who worries constantly whether everything has been done, who constantly examines the kitchens for dirt, who is forever checking the ward medicine cards lest some pills have gone astray, can soon produce a state of paralysis where all energies are taken up on checking activities while everyone forgets the real reason for the existence of the organization – the needs of the patients.

These are four areas of personality operation which seem particularly important in the doctor preparing to be an administrative therapist. Lest it may seem that he must be all virtues, it may be worth mentioning that there are a few qualities important in other fields of medicine that do not seem to matter greatly in administrative therapy. Examination ability, as shown by many degrees and diplomas, which is necessary for success in academic medicine, is of little relevance. High intelligence, critical ability, and the power to formulate ideas with incisive clarity, so necessary for scientific medical work, though useful attributes do not seem essential. Manual dexterity, necessary for major (and minor) surgery, is irrelevant. Physical toughness and the ability to function adequately at all hours of day and night, so valuable to the general practitioner, are not of great importance. Sustained energy and unrelenting ambition such as are needed for success in consulting practice are not required.

Barton[4] has suggested that it is of importance for a psychiatrist to have the appearance of a good citizen – to be happily married, to have a family, to go to church regularly. This is arguable; it may be an advantage to an administrative therapist not to be assailable on the grounds of oddity, but consideration of some of the successful administrative therapists suggests that, desirable though the public virtues may be, they are not essential to administrative therapists, and that there is room for the eccentric or unusual person.

In general, therefore, it can be said that any doctor of average abilities can become an administrative therapist provided that he has an open, responsive, spontaneous personality, a genuine regard for people, and a desire to see them develop independence and initiative. The people that will have grave difficulty in filling the role are the cynical and the manipulative, the egocentric, and the selfish, the intensely ambitious, the anxious and insecure, the rigid to whom their professional status is all-important, the suspicious and the frightened, the cold and overly scientific.

How is a doctor to obtain training as an administrative therapist? The process has hitherto been haphazard. Many of the better practitioners came to it by accident. As psychiatrists we learn to look at motivation. Why does anyone wish to become an administrative therapist? The pioneers often had an intense motivation, especially a strong identification with the patients in their suffering and their outcast, disregarded state. We must hope that there will always be others who feel this way. But a desire to study social psychiatry is also realistic: this is a most interesting field in which discoveries are being made; in the coming decades there will be many openings for people skilled in administrative therapy. It is likely that in due course the psychiatrist without some competence in administrative therapy will find it difficult to act as a senior psychiatrist in hospital, or even to gain a post. Compassion, interest in a developing field, and realistic self-interest are sound motives. A crusading desire to overthrow the established order has often mellowed into great administrative skill in many fields, though it may cause pain in early years.

Jones and Rapoport[32] gave attention to training. At the time of the study, the Belmont Unit was a pioneer one, and attracted interested doctors from all over the world. It was, however, a very unusual culture and many of them found it disturbing. They examined this 'culture shock'. The doctor had to give up wearing a uniform or a white coat, was called by his Christian name, was asked direct and personal questions by staff and patients, and had his comments or interpretations discussed, criticized, and at times rejected. This always upset the doctors; Jones and Rapoport said that it was even an advantage for a new doctor to be noticeably upset – it made him more acceptable in the unit; one of the unit's slogans was, 'We are all patients here together', and he was proving it. They pointed out, too, that the adjustment to the unit had to be more total than that which the usual hospital demands. There, any doctor will fit unless he is very odd, but 'in the unit, a doctor who does not make himself part of the unit community, become socialized to its norms and way of life and adopt a leadership position within it, cannot perform in his professional role'. They noticed that most doctors went through a period of passive observation with a certain amount of confusion, distress, and anxiety, then a period in which they tried out various ways of personal functioning until they settled down to a mode of behaviour that suited them and was acceptable to the unit. They comment that the most important area of readjustment for doctors is that of authority-responsibility, as this was so different in the unit from what doctors had learned during their professional training and experience. They almost seem to welcome these disturbances, just as analysts may welcome signs of personality disturbance as an indication that defences against anxiety are being abandoned. There is no question that for some people to acquire new modes of personal operation some disorganization of previous patterns (which produces anxiety) is necessary. But much teaching can be done without disorganizing people, and if anxiety and insecurity are too marked, little learning can occur. It seems that greater structuring of the learning process might make it more effective.

Some of these difficulties are seen elsewhere. The average mental hospital therapeutic community does not offer the entering doctor such a severe contrast as the Belmont Unit did. The abolition of titles, uniforms and personal distinctions is likely to be less marked, and the rest of the hospital retains many of the trappings with which he is familiar. But the difference is there, and the period of readjustment always takes some months.

Jones[31] has said that the only way to learn social psychiatry is to become a member of a therapeutic community. At the present time many have to learn administrative therapy by themselves, on the job, but in future it should be possible to plan training. A gradual introduction seems best; junior psychiatrists in training, internes, or, even better, medical students can sit in on ward meetings and the subsequent staff meetings as observers, preferably over a number of weeks. This introduces them to the culture; they can see other doctors operating without being in any authority themselves. Even as visitors, of course, they find the patients asking them questions, drawing them in, and using them in authority conflicts. This is a good time to do some background reading. To take charge of a small patient group or even a committee gives some experience of group-conducting. Then when the trainee comes formally on to the ward, he has a background of experience. There is still much to learn but the shock is less.

For the senior positions, of course, the best preparation is work as ward doctor of an active therapeutic community. Here the doctor can learn a more flexible way of reacting among a staff group who are almost a peer group; a group, too, who become accustomed to helping young doctors to unbuckle some of their professional armour and learn new flexibilities and sources of strength. This is the time to make experiments in modes of behaviour.

It has proved difficult to organize training for medical superintendents. Courses in medical administration tend to supply much detail about peripheral subjects – budgeting, farming, cost accounting, and organization study – and to miss out the essential skill of promoting spontaneous growth in others. These courses are not always well supported. It seems that many doctors do not care to think of themselves as potential administrators until they find themselves in an actual administrative position. It is an odd situation, rather as if they would not learn surgery until they had had to remove a few appendices or limbs; it is probably a reflection of the elaborate distaste for administrative activity inculcated by the purists of the teaching schools.

Experience in other fields, in particular management training in industry, suggests that one of the more effective ways of preparing people for new social roles, especially in administration, is to let them go away from their job for a period to study intensively with a group of others who have reached the same level. This 'release course' method has been used for generations in armies in staff college courses. On such courses men who already have knowledge and experience of their technical speciality and who are beginning to face the problems of command and management have a period of study, of instruction, and (possibly more important) of discussion and experimentation among a group of their peers. In Britain, the King Edward VII's Hospital Fund for London set up, in 1950, a Staff College for Health Service Administrators to perform this useful function, and they have run several courses for acting or potential medical superintendents. About a dozen men already working as administrators are invited for a four-week residential course; although there is substantial formal instruction by eminent and learned speakers, the main value comes from the informal discussions between the course members and their visitors, and four weeks away from their jobs is just long enough for some reflection and refocusing.

CHAPTER 7

Administrative Therapy and Other Skills

In this chapter the relationship between administrative therapy and other skills and disciplines is discussed. The indication of points of resemblance and difference serves to define administrative therapy more clearly. It shows that administrative therapy is a distinct skill; although it borrows from group psychotherapy, from business management, from hospital administration, from administrative psychiatry, and from other fields and overlaps all of them, it is both more and less than each of them.

INDIVIDUAL PSYCHOTHERAPY AND PSYCHO-ANALYSIS

The relationship between administrative therapy and individual therapy is close, as the discussion of training indicated. Administrative therapy shares most of the basic assumptions of the psychodynamic schools. Many administrative therapists have had analytic training, personal analyses, or considerable psychotherapeutic experience. Some of the early studies and many valuable experiments were carried out in institutions where most of the staff were practising analysts and many or all of the patients in individual therapy. Yet many of the principles of administrative therapy are independent of psycho-analysis, and work very similar to ours was being done by Pinel, Tuke, Conolly, and others before Freud was born.

We must acknowledge that administrative therapy owes a great deal to psychodynamic theory, as it does also to sociology and anthropology and the other social sciences. It is from these sciences that we may ultimately develop a sound theoretical basis for our work. It is probable, too, studies will continue to come from institutions where milieu therapy is combined with the intensive practice of individual therapy, such as Chestnut Lodge, McLean Hospital, the Menninger Clinic, and the Cassel Hospital. Work at such institutions, atypical though they are, has taught us a great deal of what we know about milieu therapy. It may be that there is a particular type of social system suitable to a hospital where all patients and staff are engaged in intensive individual therapy, one perhaps rather different from the system needed where the transactions are more mundane and based on work, activity, and rehabilitation. In this area there is much we have to learn, and we can hope for mutual enlightenment between individual and administrative therapy.

Inevitably, situations will develop where there will be, or seem to be, a conflict between individual and group therapy, between analytic and administrative therapy. These are usually enlargements of the inevitable clash between the needs of the individual and the group, the interests of the member and of society as a whole; at a deeper level, between the demands of the unconscious and those of external reality. At times these will be inflamed into fiery conflicts and issues of principle, especially since the proper relationship between the individual and our increasingly complex modern society is a matter of concern and personal anxiety

119

to all of us today. There is, however, no fundamental conflict between individual psychotherapy and administrative therapy; both are concerned with using psychological means to enable a disturbed individual to achieve a better balance between his internal and external life.

GROUP PSYCHOTHERAPY

Administrative therapy borrows greatly from group psychotherapy and particularly group analytic psychotherapy (see Foulkes and Anthony[23a]). The ward meeting can be regarded as a very large 'open' therapeutic group. The conducting of meetings uses very similar skills, and experience in group analytic psychotherapy is probably the best training for the administrative therapist. He will there learn to assess the movements of feeling in a meeting, the rising tension that precedes storms, the difference between the silence of calm and the silence of anger; he will become skilled at helping progress by interpretative comment. There are, however, important differences. Bion[7] pointed out the differences between a 'work' group which was organized around a common task, and analytic groups which had no task and could therefore see more clearly the unconsciously determined themes of their interaction, pairing, dependency, and fighting. The psychotherapy group has no other purpose than the analysis of the emotional disturbances of its members; they are strangers to one another, who meet only for their weekly sessions, so they can talk about things they could not mention to those they live with. The ward meeting consists of people who are living together; they have many interactions, quarrels, and excitements outside the group. Anything said in the meeting may repercuss on their daily lives. This means that no great degree of intensity or privacy of discussion can or should develop. In a community hospital, where the patients may well come from the same village or suburb, other persons' privacy may be involved, and one of the conductor's tasks may be to protect people from exposing, in an excess of frankness, material that they may later be dismayed to find common knowledge in their village. The discussion at a ward meeting is more often synthetic than analytic, more often concerned with common projects and tasks than with the unravelling of individuals' feelings. In wards where most of the patients have schizophrenic defects, it may be best, as the Cummings[18] suggest, to keep the discussion fairly firmly anchored to concrete comprehensible subjects.

The staff groups in which the administrative therapist spends much of his time are even more definitely work groups. Except in very sophisticated groups, analytic comment is out of place; in a group unaccustomed to psychodynamic talk, it may be strongly resented. It is useful to realize that a meeting of charge nurses are becoming anxious and hostile and are looking for a scapegoat on whom to vent their fury; it may be unwise to tell them so. They will merely regard the administrative therapist as a smart-alec psychiatrist and vent their fury on him! The skills and understandings of the group therapist are very useful to the administrative therapist, but he should not always display them.

There is no conflict between group analytic psychotherapy and administrative therapy. In his first book, Foulkes[23] describes activities which we should class as administrative therapy. But there is a need for the administrative therapist to consider what kind of activity each group in which he sits requires of him. In some he may be needed to act as a group therapist, offering interpretations, allowing members of the group to explore their unconsciously motivated differences and to examine the ebb and flow of emotional feeling and to analyse and re-evaluate their roles. In others there may be a job of work to do and open clashes of interest to be mediated, and the meeting's need may be for a firm, fair, and vigorous chairman who sticks to the agenda, abides by the rules of procedure, and gets through the business.

SMALL GROUP LEADERSHIP

In the last thirty years, social psychologists have amassed a good deal of experimental knowledge about small group leadership, particularly Kurt Lewin and his school.[33] This knowledge was used in Britain during the war to select potential junior officers at the War Office Selection Boards and has been used since then by industry and government. The administrative therapist should know of this theoretical work and the practical lessons that come from it, because it will inform his practice, particularly in leading work groups of staff. An example of such lessons is the often demonstrated observation that a group works much more vigorously on a plan they have drawn up themselves. If an administrative therapist knows the problem facing a forthcoming meeting, he may well be able to devise a solution. He would be unwise to announce this at the beginning of the meeting. His best course is to lay the problem before the meeting and let them work on it. It may be that they will work out a better plan than his – that is best; probably someone will come up with a plan like his which he can then agree with; only if they are stuck should he offer his plan. Then he has treated them as responsible persons capable of solving problems rather than belittling them by calling them together merely to endorse his solution.

These and many other group leadership procedures are

constantly needed in administrative therapy. The trumpeting of a ringing slogan, the public affirmation of the high ideals being served, or the raising of the spectre of an external enemy are all at times legitimate devices for strengthening the internal bonds of a group.

In working with a group of hospital officers or heads of departments, a medical superintendent can do much to set attitudes towards the inevitable and frequent problems that arise. This establishes an atmosphere among this group which will affect the whole hospital and ultimately the life of the patients. The descent of the Government Auditors can be viewed with the apprehensive resignation of the Middle Eastern peasant overwhelmed by a horde of locusts or with the zeal of a well-armed merchantman preparing to beat off a boarding attack by pirates. The first attitude is linked with the passive, defensive, apologetic custodialism of the past which made the patients into institutionalized cabbages, the second with the vigorous therapeutic optimism which leads to rehabilitation and discharges.

All these devices are legitimate and at times necessary, but administrative therapists should not forget that the primary aim is not to produce a 'happy ship' but to refit crippled people for outside life; to analyse the causes of a difference between the head nurse and the engineer and to see why they behaved as they did may be far more valuable than to gloss it over to preserve a façade of 'happiness'. This will set a pattern of problem-solving by discussion, exploration of difficulties and anxieties, and respect for the other's dignity and needs that will finally percolate all through the hospital.

MILITARY LEADERSHIP

Armies offer the most dramatic example of the leadership

of men by other men. Our history and our folklore are full of tales of charismatic leadership, of forlorn hopes and mighty warlords – Caesar, Alexander, Robert Bruce, King Alfred, Napoleon, Washington, Lincoln, and Churchill – all men with a vision or a personal sense of destiny who bound others to them, changed them and changed the world. We are all of us captives of the myths of our own culture and the assumptions about leadership which they contain. However much we may have revolted against the Carlylean concept of the world-changing hero, these tales are part of our life, with their implicit message of the power of charismatic leadership. As a result, analogies and similes drawn from the military world are constantly imported into discussions of hospital matters, especially to justify authoritarian procedures. 'You can only have one captain if you want a happy ship' is an oft-quoted tag from naval experience. These statements have an attractive simplicity and appeal to those who have happy memories of their military days – or those who are guilty because they never wore uniform.

Military service has been the lot of many in recent years; many of those in senior hospital positions in the 1960s were in uniform in World War II. Many doctors and most psychiatrists recall it with distaste; this is perhaps a fortunate antidote to military anecdotes.

The relevance of military models to administrative therapy should, however, be examined on other grounds than nostalgia or prejudice. Some lessons from military experience, particularly those common to all small group leadership, are relevant, such as the demoralizing effect of vacillating or weak leadership in an anxious time, the value of clear and explicit instructions, the invigorating and unifying effect of the enunciation of a clearly defined and

124

attainable group task. The military model of command and decision-making does not, however, fit the needs of psychiatry in many important ways. The military organization, particularly in its lower ranks, stresses uniformity and interchangeability; every sergeant must be able to do any sergeant's job. This is sensible, because individuals will be killed and wounded, and the organization must be able to go on. But it is irrelevant to civilian and hospital affairs. There is no need for every junior doctor and every charge nurse to be interchangeable at short notice with all others. As we have shown, the development of an individual style of reaction and behaviour offers the greatest therapeutic possibilities for the patients' recovery. Although there may be certain advantages in uniformity in some vast civilian bureaucracies, in the psychiatric hospital it is harmful and antitherapeutic.

The military chain of command is organized to make possible quick co-ordinated action by many people in a rapidly changing situation. There must be rapid flow of information upwards to one man equipped to decide, and rapid unquestioning obedience downwards. The social system of a ship near shore shows this clearly; the lookouts, the radar operator, the engineer all feed their information in to the captain; the helmsman and the engineer respond at once to his orders; if a rock is seen, the ship is turned aside immediately. But this is irrelevant to hospital life. There is no call for sudden, concerted action, and the rigid authoritarian hierarchy necessary to provide it is severely crippling to staff initiative and patient spontaneity. The social system of communication and authority required to support a therapeutic milieu is quite different.

For these reasons, therefore, military analogies should be used with hesitation and their precise relevance examined.

125

However, like any stock of proverbs, there are some to suit both sides in any argument and they are often handy tools to turn a corner in debate.

BUSINESS ADMINISTRATION

An administrative therapist, particularly in the post of medical superintendent, will feel that he ought to know more about business administration. A hospital resembles a business organization in some ways. It has a number of specialized departments with special needs and problems; there are a large group of employees of many different trades and skills, with their ·trade union, craft, and professional standards, checks, and balances; it consumes great quantities of supplies which have to be purchased, delivered, and controlled; it handles large amounts of money which must be controlled, audited, budgeted, and estimated. Much of the knowledge, experience, and machinery developed in the business world is clearly relevant here.

Modern business practice contributes to hospital administration in the details and mechanical minutiae of business practice and in its contributions to social system theory. The details of business practice are not relevant to the essential task of administrative therapy – that of producing an atmosphere in which patients regain social capacities – but they often show ways of doing things more effectively, and just as typewriters have taken the places of scribes, so computing machines will take the place of storemen and ordering clerks. An administrative therapist will have to know something of these things, as he will of all the other crafts with which he has marginal contact such as catering, engineering, farming, and architecture.

The medical superintendent who models himself on the business tycoon, however, may go far astray. The typical

126

business, a concern producing goods for profit, is a poor model for a hospital which does not produce goods and shows no economic profit. In a business the proper measure of efficiency is economic; does it show a profit? The finance department provides the tools to measure all the others. In a hospital there is no trading, no profit, and no economic measure. Its efficiency is most difficult to assess but can be related only to effective treatment. The use of financial measurements of efficiency in hospitals may do great harm, and it may be the administrative therapist's task to resist them and the assumptions upon which they are based. Though he may be able to learn something from studies of organizations, especially service, nonproducing organizations, the less he concerns himself with economic thinking the better. There are other people, hospital secretaries, business managers, treasurers, and finance officers, who will be very ready to work out the cost of every new project; the doctor's task is to assess their therapeutic merits and to press vigorously for the best of them. Some of the worst superintendents have been those who have become captives of their budgets, thinking constantly of the monetary cost of every project; they spread an attitude of frightened niggling throughout the hospital.

Books regarding business organization, however, are of theoretical and practical value to the administrative therapist. He will be able to see many resemblances and be given cause to reflect on his organization and methods. Several of the most useful are listed in the Reading List on p. 151.

HOSPITAL ADMINISTRATION

The hospital has to be run so that adequate supplies reach the patients and staff at the right times – enough food, clothes, pay, drugs, or tendon hammers. The organization of this, as Crocket[16] has pointed out, is 'supportive administration' and does not require a medical degree. It is, in fact, wasteful to use doctors to carry out the routine administration of hospitals and this is better done by trained laymen. In a psychiatric hospital, however, nearly all matters of administration touch on the life of the patients, and the administrative therapist, at ward or hospital level, may find himself involved.

Any attempt to rearrange the life of the patients comes into contact, and conflict, with those people already involved in running it. Though many of these are colleagues in professions linked to medicine and traditionally 'under medical direction' – nursing, occupational therapy, social work, etc. – others are not – cooking, engineering, supplies, accountancy. The administrative therapist's relationships to these people will cause him much thought, and probably much pain, grief, and fury. Many a ward doctor has retired bitterly from an encounter with an engineer, head cook, or hospital secretary, smarting from his defeat and muttering, 'You can't beat the Machine!' In an early paper, the Cummings[17] gave expression to some of these reflections in sociological terms. When a doctor becomes a medical superintendent he has to come to terms with the relationship between medical and lay administration. Some are overwhelmed and withdraw entirely. Others are challenged and interested by this new field; if appointed as medical superintendent, they plunge in, study extensively, and become 'experts' in some field of the hospital's business; they draw up the budget, plan new buildings, do their own engineering surveys, or become enthusiastic pig-breeders or dairy managers. In the spacious days of the nineteenth century, there was probably time for this. Medical superintendents planned new hospitals without benefit of architect; others ran the hospital dairy herd and won prizes at the shows; often there was insufficient money to hire a competent expert to manage the department and the Committee of Visitors were happy to have the doctor do it for them. Now there is no excuse for this. All hospital departments – engineering, catering, budgeting, supplies – call for complex skills and a knowledge of modern practices and are best left to the experts. Administrative therapy is a full-time task, and the doctor should concentrate on this.

Hospital administration today is a field of strong controversy and vigorous pressure groups. A profession of hospital administrators is well established. A group of skilled, well-trained, devoted men run the general hospitals and have established a satisfactory relationship with the general nurses and the surgeons and physicians, by which they take care of all the housekeeping, accounting, and personnel problems of the hospital. This arrangement works well, and they cannot see why it should not apply in mental hospitals. Some of them are active to 'liberate' the lay administrators in psychiatric hospitals whom they believe to be chafing under the domination of interfering and bumbling medical superintendents. They constantly press for a change; they say that they would be happy to 'free the doctors for the work for which they are trained'; they are little impressed by statements that the psychiatric hospital is quite different from a general hospital, that the way in which the patient lives is an essential part of his treatment, and that it is essential that the doctor should have control over this. They are happy to find allies in some voluble clinical psychiatrists who would also like, for entirely other reasons, to see medical superintendents abolished.

This controversy surges intermittently through British

and American psychiatry. The heat which it engenders suggests that many of the contestants are activated by self-interest – the desire to protect their job, or their self-image as essential and benevolent people – rather than the objective establishment of facts. Observation of many hospitals suggest that there are good and bad results from both systems. There are excellent psychiatric hospitals with lay governors and there are lamentable ones; there are outstanding hospitals with doctors in sole charge and there are appalling ones. Much depends on the quality of the men themselves, but even more on the political system which appoints and controls them. When the senior posts in the state mental hospitals are the principal rewards that a state governor can give to his political backers and friends, it matters little whether his duck-shooting, whisky-drinking doctor crony is made medical director or whether his incompetent and corrupt cousin is appointed administrator; either way, the patients suffer.

At the present time patterns of medical and lay responsibility vary. In most of the United States the medical superintendent has supreme authority over the hospital and is responsible for all departments – even to having to make good from his own pocket the thefts of an embezzling finance clerk. In some states (e.g. Minnesota) there are independent responsible business managers. In Britain the lay officers have been directly responsible to the Hospital Management Committee since 1948.

Whatever the particular pattern, the doctor who attempts to do administrative therapy from the medical superintendent's position will find himself with lay colleagues, skilled in their various professions, of long experience in the hospital, and secure in their competence and their position. He may have formal authority over them or he may not. Even if they are nominally subordinate to him, their knowledge of their own profession and their own department will make it difficult for him to direct them to do anything they do not agree with.

Doctors react differently to this situation. Some spend much time and effort learning the skills of others – engineering, accounting, farming – in order to direct them with knowledge. Others abdicate, overwhelmed by the technical jargon or the superior manipulative power of a lay officer, and take no interest in what happens in the department. Either extreme is unsatisfactory. The expert should run his department, but it is part of the hospital and its relationships, attitudes, and expectations affect the staff and patients in it and in contact with it. In the relations with senior officers, therefore, some of the principles of administrative therapy are most relevant. Whether or not he holds power over them, the doctor's aim should be to keep the overriding task – the welfare of the patients – before them, and to give them every opportunity to grow in their jobs. He will want to know about hospital administration, without involving himself in its minutiae. He will have to work out, over the months and years, relationships with his senior lay colleagues to enable them all to work together for the patients. He must learn enough of their jobs – the jargon, the professional and ethical standards, the permissible levities – to talk with them and to understand their problems, but he should avoid the temptation, as with anyone else in the hospital, to try to take over their jobs. He does them – and the hospital – a disservice if he tries to take their jobs, or if he spends his time trying to catch them out in minor faults. There is no need for the doctor to go seeking for peculation or pilfering in the stores or the kitchen. If the communication system is open, anything that is causing discomfort to the patients

K   131 will come to light and can be worked on. It is the task of auditors or of the police to uncover crime.

At an English mental hospital there was a cold spell just before Christmas. The elderly patients suffered considerable distress because there was not enough fuel to put on the fires. Accusations flew back and forth. The matron said that the engineer had mismanaged the coal supplies; the engineer said that the supplies officer had not ordered enough coal; the supplies officer said that the system of delivering coal had been changed and that the secretary had not told him it was not working; the secretary said that the matron failed to exercise adequate control of the use of fuel; Management Committee members who saw the old ladies shivering said that the medical superintendent was at fault in allowing this to happen. Brief inquiry established that this had happened during several previous winters and that there was a history of troubles going back at least twenty years. The medical superintendent decided that he must involve himself.

He called a meeting of all the officers and after a period of ventilation of accusations and mutual fury they began to try to find out what did happen. It soon emerged that no officer accepted responsibility, and no one really knew what was happening. During the war the engineer had been in charge of all coal and its allocation, but when rationing ceased he no longer felt himself responsible; with the appointment of a supplies officer, the secretary did not feel himself responsible; since the supplies officer had a distant office he expected that someone closer would see to it, and so on. Investigation showed that house coal was delivered from the colliery by lorry at intervals depending on the convenience of the supplier; that the coal was put in an open dump and later moved into small dumps near the wards by a ward orderly and a gang of patients with wheelbarrows. These dumps were also open and the ward staff sent patients to get as much coal as they could whenever they felt the need. There was no check of the amounts moved; the orderly just did his best to keep everyone happy. If the weather changed unexpectedly, everyone went cold.

It took five months of meetings, investigations, and checks, and several meetings with the chairman of the Management Committee, before the system of ordering was changed and the responsibilities of the various officers delineated. During this period the medical superintendent acted as chairman of the *ad hoc* committees, and he was constantly concerned with coal, its prices and qualities, until methods of supply and control had been worked out. By that time the winter was over, but in following winters supplies flowed well. The medical superintendent never again concerned himself with details of coal.

This shows the relationship of the administrative therapist to non-medical matters. These are usually the concern of the lay officers and the medical superintendent has no direct business with them. In this case, because of an unsatisfactory division of lay administrative responsibilities (ordained from above and not easy to change), the memories of ancient feuds, individual inadequacies, and personal antipathies, the organization had failed, and the patients were suffering. Each officer regretted the patients' discomfort but felt the responsibility was someone else's. It was the administrative therapist's task to bring them together, to help them to see it as a common problem and responsibility, and to work through to a solution. It was not directly the doctor's job to allocate coal, but there was nobody else available to do it at the time and so he did.

ADMINISTRATIVE PSYCHIATRY

Administrative therapy is the art of treating psychiatric patients in an institution by administrative means. As we have shown, it is best practised at the ward level; it is patient-centred and aims at rehabilitation. Administrative psychiatry is the organization of psychiatric services. It touches many fields of knowledge outside medicine – accounting, business management, law, government, health service procedure, architecture, furnishings and supplies, and often skills like laundry management, pig-breeding, and sewage disposal. It is often, alas, budget-centred. The two fields may overlap, but do not coincide. Commissioners of mental hygiene and regional psychiatrists are psychiatric administrators. Some psychiatric administrators practice administrative therapy; many do not. Some medical superintendents esteemed by state governors or regional hospital boards as 'good psychiatric administrators' because of the tidiness of their budgets and the magnificence of their new buildings or their grounds are very poor administrative therapists, running tightly organized, punitively controlled hospitals where all staff and patients go in fear and the possibilities of personal growth or rehabilitation are slight. Many of the best administrative therapists are regarded by those higher up in the organization as tiresome fellows whose requests always come at the wrong time, who never seem to know what they will want ten years from now, whose units are untidy and staff undisciplined.

Administrative psychiatry is a necessary and important task. Someone must concern himself with getting the right sort of buildings in the right place; for getting funds diverted to outpatient clinics rather than sewage farms; for planning the kinds of furniture and staff and food needed for new institutions. Much of this must be done by trained psychiatrists, since they alone have first-hand knowledge of the needs of patient and staff and they must further acquire an understanding of the world of architects, accountants, budget planners, and politicians and learn how to carry conviction to elected representatives of the people. The United States is pouring millions of dollars into mental health services, and Britain is radically altering the planning and organization of health services. In all this the guidance of skilled psychiatrists is essential. They cannot entirely prevent blunders, but some of the ghastly mistakes of the past can be avoided. These men will have to spend many hours planning, listening, talking with architects, accountants, and legislators.

OTHER SKILLS AND DISCIPLINES

There are many other fields from which the administrative therapist can learn. In some ways a psychiatric hospital is a school – a school for social learning. Some of the experience of school teachers, and especially head teachers, is relevant to administrative therapy. The work of schools for the delinquent and the disordered child is of course very similar to that of the therapeutic community and draws on the same concepts.

In his work with medical committees and even more with elected representatives in Management Committees, Regional Boards, and State Legislatures, he is entering what C. P. Snow called 'the corridors of power' – the world of politics – and he will find that some of the experiences, practices, and attitudes are relevant to his work. He will see what an effective instrument of action a committee can be when served by a really skilled chairman and how men divided by deep personal, class, and religious antipathies can be constrained by the rules of debate to work for the common good.

There are many other fields of skill that touch on administrative therapy, but they are not directly relevant to it, as are those skills discussed in this chapter.

CHAPTER 8

Theory and Results

This is a practical book suggesting types of social action doctors can take. It would be gratifying if one could point to a well-accepted body of theory justifying this social action and indubitable results forthcoming from it. But this is not possible. The doctor in a psychiatric hospital can choose only between doing administrative therapy well or badly, by accepting the challenge and responsibilities of his situation or ignoring them. His action or his inaction affects the lives of his patients. If he acts wisely he helps them greatly. If he refuses to act, and takes no interest in their lives, he abdicates as much as a surgeon who walks out in the middle of an operation. Someone else, probably uninformed, will take over the running of the patients' lives – the nurses or the lay administrative staff – and the result is most likely to be a custodial antitherapeutic milieu such as we knew in the past.

This book, therefore, is a book of recipes, not of dietetics. But this lack of a fully worked-out theoretical basis is in the tradition of medicine. Ancient medicine was hidebound by theories – the planets, the humours, the gods, the saints. From Egyptian and Chaldean times to the Middle Ages, doctors approached their patients through a fog of authority and theories of universal application. Only the Greeks for a brief time looked at what they saw and what they did, and what happened, and described this. Only in the last few centuries have doctors once again written down what they saw, what they felt, what they did and what happened, and then gone on to theorize. Now in these 'scientific' days there has been a tendency to return to theorizing and to feel that all action must await theory. In the field of social action we have insufficient theory, and empiricism offers the best guide. For twenty years doctors have been active in administrative therapy. But it is only quite recently that there has been an attempt to build a coherent theoretical framework. We need theory in three areas – we need a coherent theory of the functioning of the damaged mind, a theory of rehabilitation, and a theory of social systems and action.

THEORY

Psychological theory has given much attention to how the normal mind functions, learns, and breaks down, but not much to how it restitutes itself. Psychodynamic theory in particular has been mostly concerned with the malfunction of the mind – how its functioning goes wrong, how it breaks down, how the irrational intrudes on the rational. Freud gave attention to the functions of the ego, but his main concern was with the destructive, regressive forces. Anna Freud studied ego-function, and others have taken this further, notably Heinz Hartmann. More recently, as we have begun to understand the effects of his culture on the individual, and the social psychological approaches have begun to be integrated. The writings of Erikson are a notable example. We are beginning to have a construct of how the ego develops, and how the personality potentials of an individual interlock with the role possibilities offered by his culture. There are, however, many conceptual patterns in this field and, although no one has yet devised a satisfactory framework into which all human variations will fit, it is possible to construct a working model.

We possess a fairly adequate working model of the psychodynamics of the 'normal' individual and the person with psychoneurotic disturbance which enables us to understand them and to treat them in individual psychotherapy. The signs and symptoms of acute schizophrenia are well known and extensively studied. There has however not been much study of the psychology of chronic schizophrenics – the bulk of the long-stay mental hospital population – particularly of those factors aiding their recovery.

Even in the simpler field of physical disabilities there have been few psychodynamic studies of the factors making for recovery. Why does one man recreate a full, active, and fruitful life after losing a leg while another becomes a permanent invalid? The successful rehabilitators are usually men of drive and enthusiasm, men of faith and hope who inspire their charges. They speak of good previous personality, of personal resources, of intelligence, flexibility, and maturity, of an enduring religious faith. But they seldom give us a psychodynamic rationale for their operations. When they do, as in the writings of Aichhorn or Neill, the impression is that it was the therapist's powerful personality and immense compassion that were more important than his beliefs.

In most of the literature about milieu therapy and psychiatric rehabilitation the same lack exists. Some writers start off with theoretical suppositions which are painfully self-evident, proceed to apply remedies which have no clear connection with the suppositions, and then claim striking improvements.

Administrative Therapy

One of the best accounts of a highly successful rehabilitation programme for long-stay hospital patients – a programme intensively studied in careful detail and most fully and adequately reported – has this to say about the assumptions of the work.

'We see then that the atmosphere in which rehabilitation and therapeutic work with hard-to-reach patients can develop, requires a sense of trust and commitment, realistic goals and optimism, and a compassionate concern. It has struck us quite forcibly that these essentials in the atmosphere are none other than our old friends Faith, Hope and Charity.'[14]

Freeman, Cameron, and McGhie[24] have recently made an attempt to provide a theoretical basis for the milieu therapy of chronic schizophrenia based on Freud's and Federn's psychodynamic formulations. Their basic tenet is that the condition of schizophrenia is one in which the normal continuum between the ego and the outside world is grossly disturbed. They had a small intensive treatment centre where a few chronic schizophrenic patients spent many months in simple activities in close contact with carefully chosen staff so that durable relationships could be formed. The patients in this small therapeutic community improved markedly, but more important, the authors felt that they had confirmed their theoretical formulation.

The most comprehensive attempt to study milieu therapy and the theory behind it has been made by John and Elaine Cumming.[18] After a number of years of organizing therapeutic communities and of visiting rehabilitation hospitals they have drawn their conclusions together. In the latter half of their book they put together recommenda-

140

tions for the organization of a therapeutic milieu which are among the clearest available and their book is an essential handbook. They also touch briefly, but succinctly and rewardingly on the central concern of this book, the doctor's role in milieu therapy.

In the first section of their book they attempt to derive a psychological basis for the milieu therapy they describe. They point out that this must first be based on ego-psychology, a statement of the organism's method of interacting with its environment. They draw on the formulations of Hartmann, Erikson, Lewin, Federn, Mead, and Parsons. From these they construct a picture of ego-disorganization and a pattern of ego-restitution through milieu therapy. They say finally:

'Ego restitution may involve reorganization, redifferentiation, restitution of lost sets, addition of new sets, or set rehierarchization. In order to enable these things to happen, the milieu must offer to the patient a clear organized and unambiguous social structure, problems to solve in protected situations, and a variety of settings in which to solve these problems. It should also offer him a peer group and a helpful staff to encourage and assist him to live more effectively.'

They suggest that one of the most valuable components of the doctor's work in milieu therapy (which we have been discussing in this book) is in his effect on those nearest to the patient. By discussion, understanding, and the feeding of information he makes their response to the patient's acts more positive and less wooden, thus giving a better chance for learning to occur.

Their book is of great value and is a beginning towards

a theory of rehabilitation as a basis for our work. With such work and the many patient studies of the effects of milieu change, we may gradually obtain a theory and a body of practice generally validated and accepted.

If we had an adequate theoretical formulation of the functioning of the damaged ego and its restitutive functions, and an adequate theory of rehabilitation, it might be possible to prescribe the social system that would rehabilitate chronic psychotics most effectively. It is however far too early for that, though we must hope that from attempts such as that of the Cummings this will grow. Social science has so far had only limited success in prescribing social systems; the greatest contributions have been in demonstrating the ill effects of present institutions or the inevitability of certain developments. From all these hints the pragmatic mixture that is administrative therapy has developed, and it is to be hoped that more studies in the coming years will clarify at least some of the puzzles and show us what sort of institutions are best for psychotics to recover in and what part doctors can play in them.

RESULTS

The results of administrative therapy are not easy to assess, because it has the nonspecificity of any method of using social forces, and applied to people suffering from chronic remitting disabilities. The only diseases where assessment of remedies is easy are those with an acute predictable course or a frequently fatal outcome; as soon as we move to diseases with a chronic remitting natural history the assessment is most difficult, since psychological factors, reactions to enthusiasm, devotion of the therapists, and so on become as important as the therapy. The history of the rise and fall of cortisone treatment of arthritis in the last twenty years is a good example. The assessment of treatment methods in the acute psychoses has been difficult enough, as the rise and fall of insulin coma therapy for schizophrenia has shown; with the chronic psychoses it is even more difficult.

The aim of administrative therapy is to harness all the nonspecific social factors in a purposive way. It is based on the proposition that the main problem of many persons in psychiatric hospitals is a social disability, a loss or disintegration of the necessary social skills for survival in human society, that this disability can be alleviated by the milieu, and that this milieu, of which the most important component is the face-to-face reactions provided for the patient by those immediately round him, can only be developed if the doctors practise carefully considered administrative therapy.

To demonstrate this unequivocally is extremely difficult, perhaps impossible, there are so many variables and many of them cannot be held constant.

It is not too difficult to demonstrate the failure of the traditional custodial mental hospital to rehabilitate those suffering from chronic psychoses. Apart from all the descriptive sociological and anthropological material quoted earlier, there are the statistical facts. The number of mental-hospital beds needed rose steadily over the last century; once a patient had become 'chronic' – i.e. remained in hospital over two years – his chances of discharge were very low; the main variation over the century was that, as hygienic standards rose, the death-rate of chronic in-patient psychotics gradually fell. The custodial mental hospital was not able to rehabilitate chronic psychotics effectively, not even as well as the moral reformers had a century earlier. Further, it gave little satisfaction to the staff that worked in it, as the recurring scandals, brutalities, inexplicable deaths, and recruitment difficulties of mental hospitals showed.

Descriptions of the effects of administrative therapy are available in the writings quoted earlier, which tell of the changes in wards and in hospitals when planning of milieu therapy was introduced, but they can be summarized.

The chronic ward, from being a place of tension and control, of idleness, apathy, and hopelessness, where patients are apathetic, hostile, withdrawn and hopeless, where un-involved staff give all their interests elsewhere, and doctors visit as little as possible, becomes a lively and exciting place.

The patients emerge as people, interacting vividly and show-ing initiative, the staff are deeply interested in their patients and their ward, and the doctor is constantly involved. New projects are undertaken, there is a swirl of activity and feeling rather than the dead apathy. Indices show a decline of violence and forms of restraint, of increased activity and work, and usually of increased discharges. In a therapeutic community admitting unit it may be possible to show a shortened length of stay as well as a decline in restraints and seclusions.

The hospital to which administrative therapy has been applied shows similar changes. The old asylum atmosphere of apathy, degradation, restraint, and violence disappears; the old sight of nameless hordes of grey-faced patients (in more recent times moonfaced and soggy with tranquil-lizers) shuffling about great dreary halls, herded by sullen staff, vanishes. There is an air of purposeful activity, personal diversity, individuality, and dignity in both patients and staff, and an atmosphere of encouragement and acceptance. There is a range of activities leading toward rehabilitation and discharge and a concentration on the prospects of and preparation for leaving hospital.

Indices of this are difficult to produce. For a century there have been arguments about the meaning and reliability of statistics from asylums, with reminders of the diverse factors, and how easy it is to manipulate them. Attempts to construct yardsticks of the 'efficiency' of hospitals have caused much fury and grief without ever evolving standards acceptable both to the hospitals commended and to those discredited, by the figures. Since 1954 the number of people in English psychiatric hospitals has been falling; more recently a modest decline has been seen in some American states. This may be due to the improved administrative practices in many hospitals but it has also been attributed to other coincidental changes, such as widespread application of tranquillizers and changing social attitudes (and laws) or to a combination of coinciding population trends. The arguments and counter-arguments of the different statisticians show how difficult it is to assess the factors leading to any change in a large population.

Measurable increases in the amount of work done and a decline in restraint, seclusion, and signs of severe withdrawal such as incontinence by day have been shown following administrative therapy to a whole hospital. A rise in the discharge rate of long-stay patients has been shown. Sometimes evidence of a better service to the community, as shown by a higher voluntary admission rate, larger numbers of patients accepted, and a higher turnover with shorter stay, can be demonstrated and correlated with new policies.

Controlled studies are gradually being made and information produced. Wing[58] has carried out studies showing that long-term schizophrenic patients in more permissive hospitals had fewer florid psychotic symptoms than those in deprived and custodial surroundings. He has also shown[57] the effect that a period of changed environment in an Industrial Rehabilitation Unit has had on a group of chronic patients compared with a similar group remaining in unchanged conditions. Such studies will slowly accumulate information for us of the measurable repeatable effects of changes of environment.

It is thus difficult to work out indices that will show the exact results and value of the doctor turning his attention to administrative therapy, but the views of those involved are surely relevant. The patients have no doubt of the advantages of a régime that gives them hope and interest instead of repression and apathy. The more articulate of the long-stay patients will often express clearly their delight in their greater freedom and activity. The staff are happy to have got away from the atmosphere of tension, potential violence, and constant interfering, nagging oversight and welcome the new opportunities, the greater freedom, and enhanced public esteem of their work. For the doctor himself the change is heartening. He is no longer the uneasy titular head of a hypocritical, corrupt organization of which he is ashamed, wondering uneasily where the next scandal will erupt, or who will attack him next; he is a member of a team of respected colleagues working together, helping one of the most neglected, despised, and pathetic groups of sick, the mentally disordered who have been cast out of society. He is once more part of medicine and the curative profession, no longer a medically qualified jailer lending his status to an organization of which he secretly disapproves.

BIBLIOGRAPHY

1. ACKNER, B., HARRIS, A. & OLDHAM, A. J. Insulin Treatment of Schizophrenia – A controlled study. *Lancet*, 1957, i, 607.
2. BAKER, A. A. Factory in a Hospital. *Lancet*, 1956, i, 278.
3. BARTON, R. *Institutional Neurosis*. J. Wright & Sons, Bristol, 1959.
4. BARTON, W. E. *Administration in Psychiatry*. C. C. Thomas, Springfield, Ill., 1962.
5. BATEMAN, J. F. & DUNHAM, H. W. The State Mental Hospital as a Specialised Community Experience. *Amer.J. Psychiat.*, 1948, **105**, 445.
6. BELKNAP, I. *Human Problems of a State Mental Hospital*. McGraw-Hill, New York, 1956.
7. BION, W. R. *Experiences in Groups*. Tavistock, London; Basic Books, New York, 1961.
8. BION, W. R. & RICKMAN, J. Intra-Group Tensions in Therapy. *Lancet*, 1943, ii, 678 (also in 7 above).
9. BOURNE, H. The Insulin Myth. *Lancet*, 1953, ii, 964.
10. CARSTAIRS, G. M., CLARK, D. H. & O'CONNOR, N. Occupational Treatment of Chronic Psychotics – Observations in Holland, Belgium and France. *Lancet*, 1955, ii, 1025.
11. CARSTAIRS, G. M., O'CONNOR, N. & RAUNSLEY, K. Organisation of a Hospital Workshop for Chronic Psychotic Patients. *Brit.J.Prev.Soc.Med.*, 1956, **10**, 136.
12. CAUDILL, W. A. *The Psychiatric Hospital as a Small Society*. Harvard University Press, Cambridge, Mass., 1958.
13. CAUDILL, W. A., REDLICH, F. C., GILMORE, H. R. & BRODY, E. B. Social Structure and Interaction Processes on a Psychiatric Ward. *Amer.J.Orthopsychiat.*, 1952, **22**, 314.
14. CHITTICK, R. A., BROOKS, G. S., IRONS, F. S. & DEANE, W. N. *The Vermont Story*. Queen City Printers, Burlington, Vermont, 1961.

Bibliography

15. CLARK, D. H. Functions of the Mental Hospital. *Lancet*, 1956, ii, 1005.
16. CROCKET, R. W. Doctors, Administrators and Therapeutic Communities. *Lancet*, 1960, ii, 359.
17. CUMMING, J. & E. The Locus of Power in the Large Mental Hospital. *Psychiatry*, 1956, **19**, 361.
18. CUMMING, J. & E. *Ego and Milieu*. Atherton Press, New York, 1962; Tavistock Publications, London, 1964.
19. DENBER, H. C. B. *Research Conference on Therapeutic Community*. C. C. Thomas, Springfield, Ill.; Blackwell, Oxford, 1960.
20. DUNHAM, W. & WEINBERG, S. K. *The Culture of the State Mental Hospital*. Wayne State University Press, Detroit,1960.
21. EARLY, D. F. The Industrial Therapy Organisation (Bristol). *Lancet*, 1960, i, 754.
22. EARLY, D. F. The Industrial Therapy Organisation (Bristol). *Lancet*, 1963, i, 435.
23. FOULKES, S. H. *Introduction to Group Analytic Psychotherapy*. Heinemann, London, 1948.
23a. FOULKES, S. H. & ANTHONY, E. J. *Group Psychotherapy—the Psycho-analytic Approach*. Penguin Books, Harmondsworth, 1957.
24. FREEMAN, T., CAMERON, J. L. & MCGHIE, A. *Chronic Schizophrenia*. Tavistock Publications, London; International Universities Press, New York, 1958.
25. GOFFMAN, E. The Characteristics of Total Institutions. *Symposium on Preventive and Social Psychiatry*, see 55.
26. GOFFMAN, E. *Asylums*. Doubleday, New York, 1961.
27. GREENBLATT, M., YORK, R. H. & BROWN, E. L. *From Custodial to Therapeutic Patient Care in Mental Hospitals*. Russell Sage Foundation, New York, 1955.
28. GREENBLATT, M., LEVINSON, D. J. & WILLIAMS, R. N. *The Patient and the Mental Hospital*. The Free Press, Glencoe, Ill., 1957.
29. JONES, M. *Social Psychiatry*. Tavistock Publications, London, 1952. Under the title *The Therapeutic Community*, Basic Books, New York. C. C. Thomas, Springfield, Ill., 1962.
30. JONES, M. *Social Psychiatry*. C. C. Thomas, Springfield, Ill., 1962.

148

31. JONES, M. Training in Social Psychiatry at Ward Level. *Amer.J.Psychiat.*, 1962, **118**, 705.
32. JONES, M. & RAPOPORT, R. N. The Absorption of New Doctors into a Therapeutic Community. In Greenblatt *et al.*, *The Patient and the Mental Hospital*, see 28 above.
33. LEWIN, K. *Field Theory in Social Science.* Harper & Bros., New York; Tavistock Publications, London, 1951.
34. MAIN, T. F. The Hospital as a Therapeutic Institution. *Bull.Menn.Clin.*, 1946, **10**, 66.
35. MAINE, H. *If a Man be Mad.* Doubleday, New York, 1947; Gollancz, London, 1952.
36. MARTIN, D. V. Institutionalization. *Lancet*, 1955, ii, 1188.
37. MARTIN, D. V. *Adventure in Psychiatry.* Cassirer, London, 1962.
38. MARTIN, D. V. *Handbook for Staff at Claybury Hospital.* 1961.
39. MYERSON, A. Theory and Principles of the 'Total Push' Method in the Treatment of Chronic Schizophrenia. *Amer.J.Psychiat.*, 1939, **95**, 1197.
40. NIGHTINGALE, F. *Notes on Hospitals – Matters affecting Health, Efficiency and Administration.* Longman, Roberts & Green, London, 1863.
41. PARKINSON, C. N. *Parkinson's Law or the Pursuit of Progress.* Murray, London, 1958.
42. PATTEMORE, J. C. The Development of a Disturbed Ward. *Nurs.Times*, 1957, Jan. 18.
43. PATTERSON, T. T. *Morale in War and Work.* Max Parrish, London, 1955.
44. RAPOPORT, R. N. *Community as Doctor.* Tavistock Publications, London, 1960; C. C. Thomas, Springfield, Ill., 1961.
45. ROGERS, C. R. *On Becoming a Person.* The Riverside Press, Cambridge, Mass., 1961.
46. ROWLAND, H. Interaction Processes in the State Mental Hospital. *Psychiatry*, 1938, **1**, 323.
47. ROWLAND, H. Friendship Patterns in the State Mental Hospital. *Psychiatry* 1939, **2**, 363.
48. SHOENBERG, E. & MORGAN, R. Starting a Schizophrenic Unit. *Lancet*, 1958, ii, 412.

Bibliography

49. SIMON, H. More Active Treatment of Mental Patients in Hospital. *Allg.Z.Psychiatr.*, 1927, **87**, 97–145, and 1929, **90**, 69–121.
50. SIVADON, P. Techniques of Sociotherapy. In *Symposium on Preventive and Social Psychiatry*, see 55 below.
51. STANTON, A. & SCHWARTZ, M. *The Mental Hospital.* Basic Books, New York, 1954.
52. SULLIVAN, H. S. *Schizophrenia as a Human Process.* W. W. Norton, New York, 1962.
53. WADSWORTH, W. V., SCOTT, R. F. & TONGE, W. L. Hospital Workshop, *Lancet*, 1958, ii, 896.
54. WADSWORTH, W. V., WELLS, B. W. P. & SCOTT, R. F. The Organisation of a Sheltered Workshop. *J. Ment.Sci.*, 1962, **108**, 780.
55. Walter Reed Army Institute of Research. *Symposium on Preventive and Social Psychiatry.* U.S. Govt. Printing Office, Washington, D.C., 1958.
56. WILMER, H. A. *Social Psychiatry in Action.* C. C. Thomas, Springfield, Ill., 1958.
57. WING, J. K. & GIDDENS, R. G. T. Industrial Rehabilitation of Male Chronic Schizophrenic Patients. *Lancet*, 1959, ii, 505.
58. WING, J. K. & BROWN, G. W. Social Treatment of Chronic Schizophrenia – A comparative study of three mental hospitals. *J.Ment.Sci.*, 1961, **107**, 847.
59. World Health Organization. Expert Committee on Mental Health, 3rd Report. Geneva, 1953.

150

READING LIST

I have had many requests for a reading list for administrative therapy, but have found it difficult to supply, for in postgraduate study everyone must find his own path, culling from those authors who make sense to him and abandoning those who do not help. This list is personal: the following are books which I found of value and I list them in the hope that others may benefit. There may well be other books as good or even better which I either failed to find or lacked the diligence to study fully. Bibliographical details of titles marked with an asterisk are given in the Bibliography.

Social Psychology
LEWIN, K. *Resolving Social Conflicts.* Harper, New York, 1948.
LEWIN, K. *Field Theory in Social Science.**
SPROTT, W. J. H. *Social Psychology.* Methuen, London, 1952.

Anthropology
BENEDICT, R. *Patterns of Culture.* Houghton Mifflin, Boston, 1934; Penguin Books, Harmondsworth, 1946.
MEAD, M. *Male and Female.* Penguin Books, Harmondsworth, 1962.
RIESMAN, D. *The Lonely Crowd.* Yale University Press, New Haven, Conn., 1950.
WHYTE, W. H. *The Organization Man.* Simon & Schuster, New York, 1956; Cape, London, 1957.

Studies of Industry
BROWNE, J. A. C. *Social Psychology of Industry.* Penguin Books, Harmondsworth, 1954
DRUCKER, P. F. *The Practice of Management.* Harper, New York, 1954; Heinemann, London, 1955.

151

Reading List

JAQUES, E. *The Changing Culture of a Factory*. Tavistock Publications, London, 1951.

MAYO, E. *The Human Problems of an Industrial Civilization*. Macmillan, New York, 1933; Routledge & Kegan Paul, London, 1949.

MCGREGOR, D. *The Human Side of Enterprise*. McGraw-Hill, New York, 1960.

PARKINSON, N. C. *Parkinson's Law.* *

URWICK, L. *The Elements of Administration*. Pitman, London, 1947.

Hospital Studies

BARTON, R. *Institutional Neurosis.* *

BELKNAP, I. *Human Problems of a State Mental Hospital.* *

CAUDILL, W. *The Psychiatric Hospital as a Small Society.* *

DUNHAM, W. & WEINBERG, S. K. *The Culture of the State Mental Hospital.* *

GREENBLATT, M., LEVINSON, D. & WILLIAMS, R. *The Patient and the Mental Hospital.* *

STANTON, A. & SCHWARTZ, M. *The Mental Hospital.* *

Walter Reed Army Institute. *Symposium on Preventive and Social Psychiatry.* *

Hospital Studies: Critical

DEUTSCH, A. *Shame of the States*. New York, Harcourt, Brace, 1948.

GOFFMAN, E. *Asylums.* *

MAINE, T. *If a Man Be Mad.* *

Hospital Studies: Fiction

GIBSON, W. *Cobweb*. Knopf, New York; Secker & Warburg, London, 1954.

KESEY, K. *One Flew over the Cuckoo's Nest*. Viking Press, New York, 1962.

WARD, M. J. *The Snake Pit*. Cassell, London, 1947.

Therapeutic Communities

GREENBLATT, M., YORK, R. H. & BROWN E. L. *From Custodial to Therapeutic Patient Care in Mental Hospitals.* *

JONES, M. *Social Psychiatry* (1952).*
JONES, M. *Social Psychiatry* (1963).*
MARTIN, D. V. *Adventure in Psychiatry.**
RAPOPORT, R. *Community as Doctor.**
WILMER, H. *Social Psychiatry in Action.**

Historical
BOND, E. *Dr. Kirkbride and His Mental Hospital.* Lippincott, Philadelphia, 1947.
BROWNE, W. A. F. *What Asylums Were, Are, and Ought to Be.* Black, Edinburgh, 1837.
CONOLLY, J. *The Treatment of the Insane without Mechanical Restraints.* Smith Elder & Co., London, 1856.
PINEL, P. *A Treatise on Insanity* (1806). Hathner Publishing Company, New York, 1962.
TUKE, S. *Description of the Retreat, York.* Alexander, York, 1813.

Theory
CUMMING, J. & E. *Ego and Milieu.**
FOULKES, S. H. & ANTHONY, E. J. *Group Psychotherapy.*
FREEMAN, T. & others. *Chronic Schizophrenia.**
SULLIVAN, H. S. *Schizophrenia as a Human Process.**

Administrative Psychiatry
BARTON, W. E. *Administration in Psychiatry.**
BRYAN, W. *Administrative Psychiatry.* Allen & Unwin, London, 1937; Norton, New York.
Group for the Advancement of Psychiatry. *Administration of the Public Mental Hospital.* New York, 1960.

INDEX

abuse, protection from, 34f
Ackner, B., Harris, A., and
Oldham, A. J., 7
activity, importance of, 40
adjustment to unit, 114
administration
relations with lay, 128
supportive, 128
admission procedures, discussion of, 72
Aichhorn, A., 139
analysis, personal, 104
anxiety, obsessional, 111ff
arthritis, cortisone treatment,
143
asylum management, basic
principles, 32ff
atmosphere of hospital, 38ff
attendants, beliefs of, 12
attitude, doctor's, to people,
107f
authority,
conflicts with, 109
examining structure, 55f
flattening of, 45f
flexibility of, 67f
sapiential and structural, 62

Baker, A. A., 17
Banstead Hospital, 17
barrier mechanics, 91
barriers, adjusting, 71f, 100
Barton, R., 14
Barton, W. E., 113
Bateman, F. J., and Dunham,
H. W., 8

bathing parade, 33f
Bedford Veterans Administration Hospital, 27
Bed Rest Treatment, 15
behaviour, aberrant, 42
Belknap, I., 11, 51
Bell, George Macdonald, 19, 93
Belmont Hospital, 25f, 91, 114
Bicêtre, 19
Bion, W. R., 120
Bion, W. R., and Rickman, J.,
24
Board of Control, 16f, 19, 38
Boston conference (1956), 28
Boston Psychopathic Hospital,
27
Bourne, H., 7
business administration, 126f

cardiazol, 5
Carstairs, G. M., Clark, D. H.,
and O'Connor, N., 17
Carstairs, G. M., O'Connor, N.,
and Raunsley, K., 17
Cassel Hospital, 119
Caudill, W. A., 11
charge nurse, in therapeutic
community, 85
Cheadle Royal Hospital, 17
Chestnut Lodge, 8, 119
child guidance clinics, 3
chronic patients, 4
Claybury Hospital, 29, 91
Columbus State Hospital, 8
Commissioners in Lunacy, 19,
38

155

Printed and bound by CPI Group (UK) Ltd, Croydon, CR0 4YY

01/11/2024

01782630-0010